Suzy Prudden's Exercise Program for Young Children

Suzy Prudden's Exercise Program for Young Children

By Suzy Prudden

Foreword by Burton L. White, Ph. D.

Photographs by Douglas Hopkins

Workman Publishing, New York

Library of Congress Cataloging in Publication Data

Prudden, Suzy.
  Suzy Prudden's Exercise program for young children.

  1. Exercise for children.   I. Title.   II. Title:
Exercise program for young children.
RJ133.P79   1983   613.7′ 1′ 088054   82-40506
ISBN 0-89480-371-9 (pbk.)

Book design by Charles Kreloff with Kathy Herlihy
Cover photograph by Stephen AuCoin
Cover wardrobe courtesy of Capezio Ballet Makers
Children's sweat suits courtesy of Morris Brothers

Workman Publishing Company, Inc.
1 West 39th Street
New York, N.Y. 10018

Manufactured in the United States of America
First printing September, 1983

10 9 8 7 6 5 4 3 2 1

Dedication:

To friends and family, all on the rainbow road to the big grok candy mountain: Steven and Kevin Silverman, June Graham and Jim Spencer, Rona Cherry, Elizabeth Brenner, Larry Weiss, Diane Terman, Martha Coopersmith, Jeanne Bacols, Imalda Collier, and Ruth Ginzberg.

To Ray Gottlieb, whose vision it is to see beyond clearly, and to Rita Silverman, who clearly sees beyond vision.

To the two most important people and best friends to me in this life: my son, Robby Sussman—at age 17 a handsome, creative, and extraordinary young man; and to my mother, Bonnie Prudden, a guiding star—a beacon of brilliance in heart and mind.

To the family Gallucci, with whom I greet and light up the world as we go with passion and ''do'' the planet.

And to the Universe, whose gifts to me I now give the babies.

Special thanks to all the children who participated in the photographing of this book:

Holly Anjer
Jeremy Basescu
Jeffrey Baumstein
Bradford Beckerman
Nicole DePalma
Kate Fiscalini
Rachel Fleischner
Jordan Fraser
Tracy Gertler
Aaron Goldsmid
Jeremy and Lauren Goldstein
Bradley Gumbel
Michael Hertzberg
Miriam Hurwitz
Shaun Jessie
Rachel Josué
Julianna Kelly

Kevin Kunstadt
Irene Longshore
Matthew Miller
Kimberley Moss
Laura Plattner
Brendon Ratner
Devin Reiter
Jessica Saar
Sara Sgobbo
Katie Shopkorn
Matthew Silberstein
Kevin Silverman
Neil Solinsky
Rachel and Stephanie Stern
Emily and Julie Turner
Justin Yadgaroff

Contents

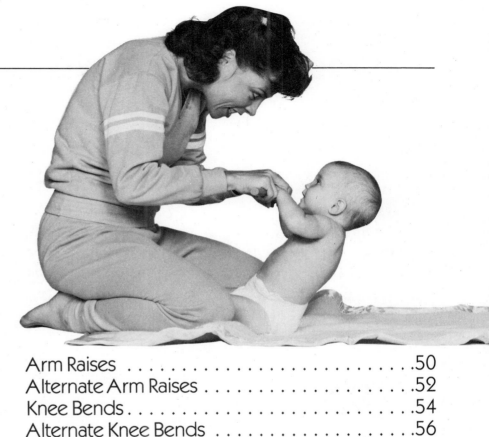

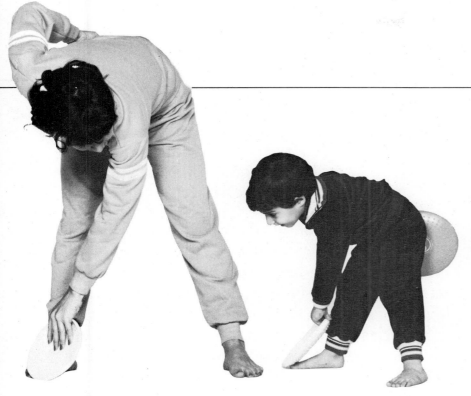

Foreword

This is a delightful, clearly written, and potentially very useful book for parents of very young children. The reason it is delightful is the author's warm style, which reflects her obvious enjoyment and love of young children. Its clarity is no doubt the result of years of writing books on this topic. The potential usefulness of the book is rooted in a fundamental fact about the healthy young child. Babies *have* to master their bodies during the first years of their lives, and the possibilities for enjoyment as well as learning are substantial. I have written elsewhere that from the time they begin to crawl about on their own, which usually is around seven months, babies have three key interests. One is the satisfaction of curiosity. The second is the person around whom their day revolves. The third is mastering their own bodies.

Parents who follow the suggestions in this book will be helping to meet at least two of their child's principal needs during the early years. They will be spending a good deal of time with their child in the activities, and second, they will be helping the child to achieve the bodily control that is very much suited to their natural tendencies. Along the way, as an added

bonus, it is highly likely that there will be a good deal of language learning because of the nature of the shared activities. Last, but not least, since these activities are likely to be very enjoyable for both parties, the relationship between parent and child is likely to be enhanced by the great fun that will be involved.

Let me say a few words about what this book is *not*. It is not a book designed to create precocious gymnastic skills in your child. Ms. Prudden, thankfully, is not a member of the group of "experts" that seeks to support efforts to create unusual early skills in young children. Indeed, if she were, I would not suggest that you use this book.

Second, this is not a book on how to raise a child. You will have to go elsewhere for that kind of information. I have some suggestions as to where you might find such information, but I am much too modest to include them here. While this is not a book on how to raise a child, it could not be a recommendable book in my eyes if Ms. Prudden were not well-informed about development in the first years of life. Ms. Prudden is indeed well-informed about the normal developments of the first years. This is reflected in the accuracy of her remarks about the development of the abilities to hold one's head erect, sit up, crawl, climb, etc. The book clearly reveals that much of this detailed information comes from extensive experience with young children. One simply could not write a book of this quality without that kind of experience.

In summary, infants, toddlers, and preschoolers *love* mastering their bodies and related motor activities. This book is full of useful, easy-to-follow information about how to help children through these stages. Following Ms. Prudden's exercises will provide not only direct benefits in body control and confidence, but lots of fun times for children as well. Its advice is consistent with what I know about how to help a child off to a good start in life, and I therefore recommend it with enthusiasm.

Burton L. White, Ph.D.
Director, Center for Parent Education
(Newton, Mass.), and author of
The First Three Years of Life and
A Parent's Guide to the First Three Years

Introduction

Children are born with bodies and minds. Since they are truly dependent in infancy, we, as parents, must offer them the best and most interesting environment and activities possible to encourage mental and physical growth.

Fancy toys will not promote an infant's motor development, because all he does at that age is stare at them. And television certainly does not activate the toddler's brain. (It doesn't activate *anyone's* brain.) But infants do respond to stimulation and repetition. It has been proven that through careful, loving handling, babies learn. A baby is like a little sponge. He* may not show it for a while, but he soaks up all you give him. And one of the most valuable things you can give a baby is exercise.

Babies who are exercised become more flexible and coordinated. They learn language, since you continually talk to them during a session. They are introduced to rhythm, since you play and move to music. They gain in muscle strength and, most important, in

---

*I use the masculine pronoun throughout this book for semantic convenience only.

self-esteem—they feel your love and therefore are happy with you and with themselves. If you offer your child new activities, he will begin to look forward to the next challenge; his curiosity is fostered. And as each new challenge is met and successfully achieved, self-confidence is born—setting up an important pattern for later in life.

Many parents feel that their child is advanced because he can sit up or roll over sooner than another. Other parents worry because their child doesn't move at the same pace as a friend's child. Parents are always comparing their children with everyone else's. But no child is "better" than another. He is simply different.

Some babies begin to talk sooner than others. But actually, babies are communicating all the time. Their conversation, although not in actual words, is nonstop. A baby communicates in many different ways without having to speak. Holding his hands up to say, "Hold me," pointing and grunting to say, "I want that," shaking his head back and forth to say, "No"—your baby is constantly "talking" to you. Pay attention to him.

Be aware, too, of how you focus on your child when he doesn't articulate well. You concentrate much harder on understanding him when he has difficulty than when things come more easily. It is important to re-member to be just as attentive when a child's actions and speech are clear as when they are unclear. If you just nod and go about your business when you under-stand what your child is trying to say, he may well go out of his way to get your attention with communica-tions that make absolutely no sense at all.

Your child can not only communicate; he can under-stand you. Think of how his face lights up when you come into the room. Then imagine how wonderful it is for him to do something and have you repeatedly respond with joy and approval. If you say "no" or "don't" all the time and you react more strongly to the negative than the positive, your child is going to sense this. If a no brings a quicker, more forceful response than a yes, rest assured that your child will go after the no.

These patterns, like movement, are established early, and will be a part of your child's life for a long time. You can make the difference by placing the emphasis on the positive.

This brings us back to fitness and exercise and the purpose of this book. Every time you exercise your baby and are happy with his progress, your baby feels this positive reaction. Every time your child learns a new physical feat and you respond with delight, your child will feel wonderful—and will strive for this response again and again. Each new challenge will be exciting, something to look forward to. And how won-derful it is to look forward to challenges rather than to be afraid of them!

Babies are constantly adding new items to their physical and intellectual vocabularies. Every time you introduce a new exercise or object, your baby needs time to absorb it and to become comfortable with it. As your baby masters each new activity and assimi-lates each new experience, he will look forward to something new. Praise and encourage him in this—even at this age.

But babies also like repetition. They feel comfortable with it. What we may find boring brings security to a child. After a baby grasps an exercise, he will want to practice it. By practice, I don't mean doing the exer-cise himself. In the case of the infant and young child, practice means Mommy or Daddy doing the exercises daily with him—and, if possible, in the same order. Practicing simple skills builds the foundation on which we add more difficult skills.

The "tricks" your child learns through exercise very often have additional safety benefits. Many parents want to know how to safety-proof their babies. In all my years as a parent and teacher, I have not found a way to protect a child completely other than by locking him up (which I do *not* recommend). We can help babies learn how to use and control their bodies—which will increase their safety. But your baby holds a thought for only seconds. One minute, he knows not to get too close to the edge of a staircase (it looks awfully high up); the next moment, he has forgotten his fear of heights and thinks it would be fun to be downstairs. Unfortunately, he sometimes makes the journey head first. So teach your child how to handle obstacles—and take suitable precautions.

One September, a client of mine returned to my studio for classes after summer with a wonderful story. Her 10-month-old son Jeremy was racing across the yard on all fours. He approached a forgotten and therefore unattended ditch. Before anyone could grab him, he was over the edge. His mother yelled, "Tuck!" and Jeremy thrust out his arms, tucked his head under, and did a perfect somersault. When hauled out of the ditch, all he had on his face—which could have been bruised—was a huge smile. He was quite pleased with himself, as he thought he had done his somersault perfectly. His mother was pleased that he had not been hurt. And a fence was put around the ditch.

Your child will grow from a passive participant to an active one as you exercise him daily. As your child begins to move, not only in place, but across the floor, you will want to add obstacles to his exercise program. A child at any stage is happy when challenged physically as well as mentally as he goes from point A to point B. Add obstacles that he can crawl over, under, around, or through, and you add new dimensions to his mental and physical fitness. As your baby becomes proficient at the exercises outlined in each section, you may go on to incorporate exercises from other sections. If he can handle more advanced movements, allow him to try them!

"Setting up simple obstacles provides input to mental growth," says Dr. Burton L. White in his book, *The*

First Three Years of Life. This is true, of course, of physical growth as well. If your baby is not yet walking, have him crawl on the equipment. But only use what your baby is comfortable with. Don't push him; guide him.

You may not realize it, but babies get tense just like adults do. Granted, these tensions are not caused by the same things. A baby's tension builds up in an inactive body. Often the only way he can release this tension is to cry (which will often create tension in you). This may explain why some children seem to cry for no reason. Through exercise, tension can be released.

Babies who are allowed to be inactive can become listless and uninterested in things around them. This can become an unfortunate pattern that may last through adult life. Take care of both tension and lethargy by encouraging your child to be active. You can accomplish this and instill good habits for life by offering him plenty of creative and beneficial exercises. "If we begin soon enough and are consistent long enough, we can help establish in our babies the habit of exercising," says Bonnie Prudden in her book, *Pain Erasure the Bonnie Prudden Way.*

It is important to realize that, although all children grow up at more or less the same rate, those offered physical and intellectual stimulation are better equipped to deal with adult life. Exercise done on a daily basis will give him a strong, balanced, coordinated, and well-formed body. A child who walks well and stands straight will grow up to be an adult who exudes strength. And your child's imagination and self-confidence will be enhanced with exercise. He will en-achieving his goals as an adult because he succeeded at the many challenges you created for him as a child.

There are no easy answers in child-rearing. There are no absolutes. We must simply give our children the best that each of us can give. This book can help you give your child that better start in life. As I stated earlier, most babies start out the same. It is up to us as parents to make the difference between a strong, vital child and a weak, unhappy one.

I do not propose to make your children supermen and women. I do propose a program that gives you the opportunity to offer your child a healthy, happy beginning. This is the strongest foundation for life that anyone can ask for.

Suzy Prudden

Baby Massage

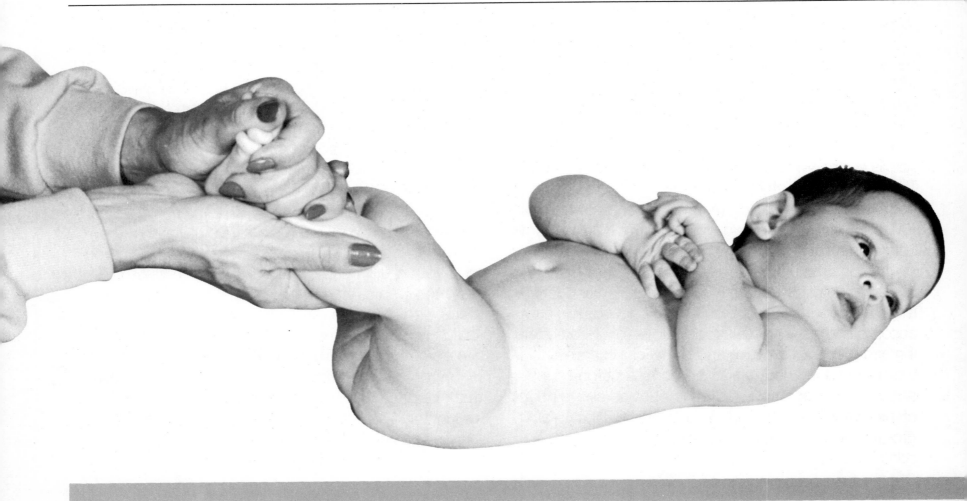

Nothing seems more vulnerable than a new-born infant. Your baby is so small and apparently fragile that you may sometimes be afraid to handle him except when you are feeding or diapering him.

But this is not enough. In addition to food, warmth, and sleep, your baby needs active love. Your child needs to be held, to be touched, to be communicated with in a way that he physically feels and therefore comprehends.

Your baby cannot understand when you tell him you love him, but he can sense it when you touch him with firm, reassuring, loving hands. By massaging your baby, you not only build your own confidence in your ability to handle your child properly—you definitely communicate messages of love and reassurance.

Touch is one of the first senses to which your baby responds. And when you touch your infant, you do more than simply send messages of love to him. Nerve endings in the baby's body react to the touch, sending a message to the spinal cord, which then forwards that message to the brain. Although we can't see it, there is actual physical change in the brain as a result of this stimulus. Not only is your baby's body growing and gaining weight; the brain's weight, protein content, and enzyme activity are increasing measurably.

Studies in hospitals have shown that babies who are handled and caressed have a higher percentage of brain growth than those who are not handled. Moreover, these babies are much more aware of what's going on around them. Babies who are touched, held, and handled often respond well to outside stimuli and become more actively aware of and responsive to all their surroundings.

A beautiful way to stimulate the brain as well as foster the feeling of love and security in your child is baby massage. Your baby's brain will register the touch of your hands, and he will also feel the different parts of his body that you place your hands on. Thus, he not only feels the warmth and love and relaxation created by massage, but also becomes aware of his limbs.

Start your massage program as soon as possible. The sooner you have more physical contact with your child, the sooner any fears you have about handling him will be alleviated. And babies love to be touched. They have no innate fears about being held. The more you touch and handle your baby, the more love he feels and the less fear you feel. You and your infant will get to know each other more quickly, and you yourself will be more comfortable and confident. Massage helps to build up the love bond between parent and child, and it helps to soothe and relax a child.

Massage is excellent for stimulating circulation in your child. The brain is fed by oxygen in the bloodstream that is circulated throughout the body. Since babies spend most of their early weeks asleep, their circulation is normally slow. By massaging your child, you speed up circulation for brief periods, energizing your infant and sending surges of fresh oxygen through the bloodstream to the brain. And massage feels wonderful. It is an activity that both parent and child can look forward to.

It is important to note here that fathers, too, should participate in their children's massage and exercise program. Daddy should never be left out. The more you offer a child in the way of physical contact, the more secure the child will become. And in some ways, fathers who massage their infants benefit even more than their children do. This is a totally new and different experience for most of them, one that can generate real tenderness and delight. The father gains confidence and security as he handles his baby and is reassured that he, too, can share in and contribute to

his child's growth.

To start your massage program, all you need is a warm room, a soft quilt, some baby oil, gentle music if possible, loving hands, and a naked baby. This is *your* time with your baby, so choose it carefully. Your baby should be alert and comfortable. It doesn't matter if it's morning, afternoon, or evening, or before or after sleep; it must simply be a pleasant and relaxed time for both of you.

The best place to do baby massage is on the floor. (I do not recommend using a bed as a massage table because it's awful for your back.) A changing table or counter may be used during the first few weeks and even months, but remember, as soon as your baby becomes active, high places are not safe. A baby has nowhere to fall when resting on the floor.

Place your baby on the quilt on his back. Take a small amount of oil in your hands. Rub your hands together to warm the oil to body temperature and, as you talk and croon to your child, begin to massage. If you tell your baby what you are doing, he will begin to process the information and store the sounds as well as the touch sensations in his brain.

I suggest doing baby massage for about 20 minutes. This may be shortened or lengthened depending on your schedule and your baby's mood. Actually, unlike exercise, massage time can run into your baby's nap time, since massage will not keep a baby from sleeping. Just be sure it is a happy, loving time. When finished, wrap your baby in a soft towel and hug.

Very often, agitated babies can be calmed by a massage. The soft music and gentle, firm stroking of the torso and limbs helps release tension and relaxes children if they are upset. The steady motion of your hands on your baby's body is reassuring. But keep in mind that the massage that calms a cranky baby should not replace the regular massage time that you and your infant spend together.

In the beginning, your baby will not move much during the massage. But there are days, as your baby advances in age, when he will twist and turn, slipping right through your fingers. When this occurs, don't force the massage. Keep it up only as long as your baby likes. Remember: we all have days when we are irritable or touchy. Respect your baby's feelings.

Chest and Tummy

When you slowly and gently stroke your baby's chest and tummy, your child's circulation will be stimulated and muscles will relax. Massaging the chest

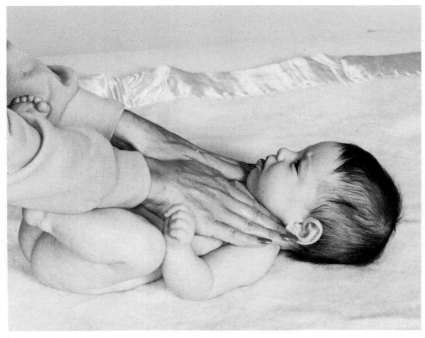

1. Place your baby on his back and put your hands on and around his shoulders.

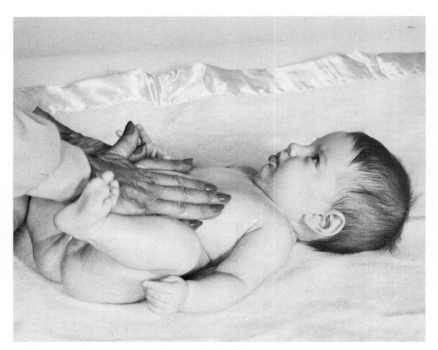

2. Slowly and gently move your hands down over your baby's chest and tummy.

and tummy stimulates internal organs
as well.

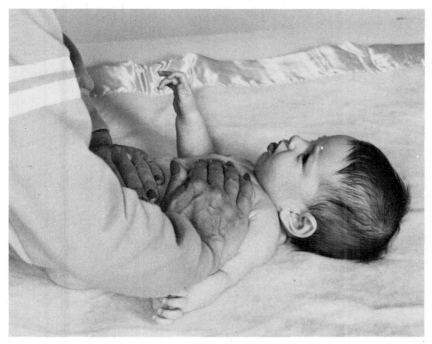

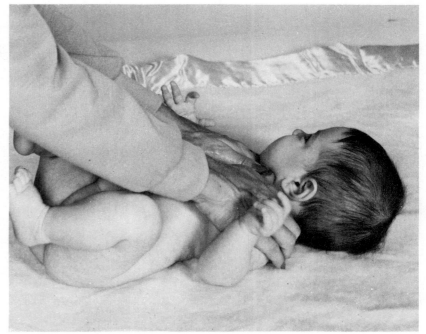

3. Turning the heels of your hands outward and your fingertips inward, slowly move your hands up across his chest.

4. When your hands have reached your baby's shoulders, reach behind his neck with your fingers and then bring your hands back down across his chest. Repeat the sequence 6 times.

Shoulders and Arms

Your baby carries tension in his shoulders just as you do. By stroking and massaging them, you release some of this tension, helping your baby to relax.

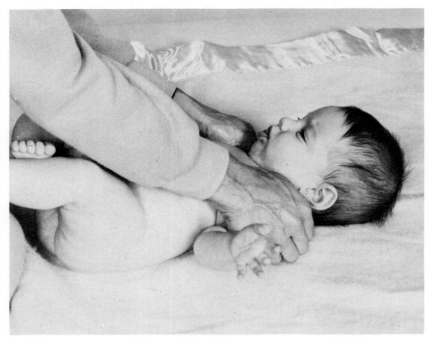

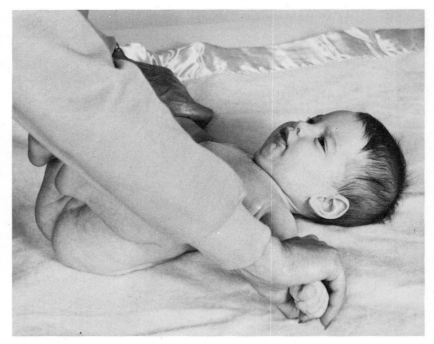

1. Place your baby on his back and clasp his shoulders gently with your hands. Slowly rub his shoulders 4 times in an outward circular motion, then 4 times in an inward circular motion.

2. Gently take hold of your baby's shoulders again. Clasping both of his arms, move your hands down his arms to his hands. Repeat this action 4 times.

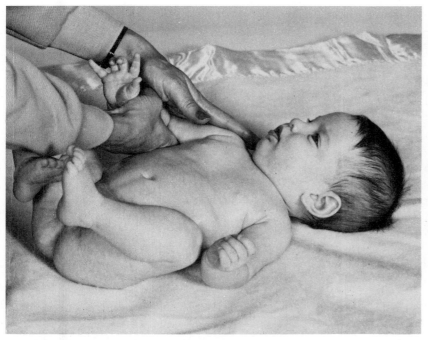

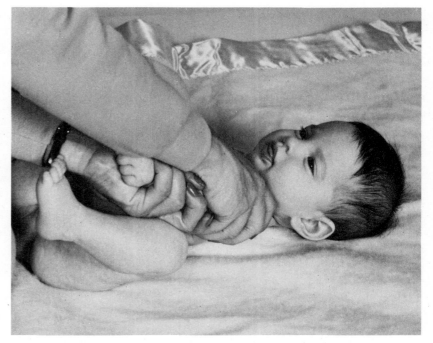

3. Then take your baby's right arm and shoulder in both of your hands, and alternating hands, stroke the inside and outside of his arm from shoulder to hand 6 times.

4. Take your baby's left arm and shoulder in both of your hands and repeat this action 6 times.

Chest and Back

By evenly massaging your baby's chest and back, you help regulate your child's breathing as well as stimulate the circulatory system.

1.

Place your baby on his back and put your hands on his chest with your fingertips wrapped around the sides of his rib cage. You will probably be able to cover his whole chest with your hands.

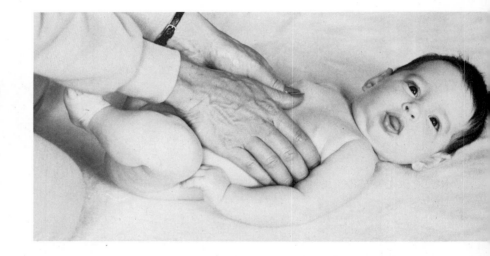

2.

Gently stroke outward, reaching your hands all the way around to your baby's back.

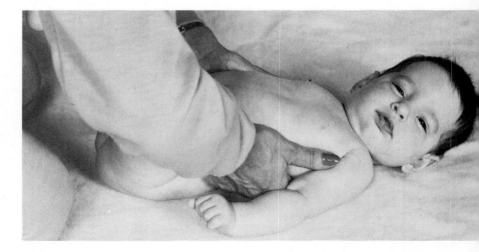

3.

Using your fingers, first press inward against your baby's back and then, bringing your hands around his chest, against the sides of his rib cage. Repeat the sequence 6 times.

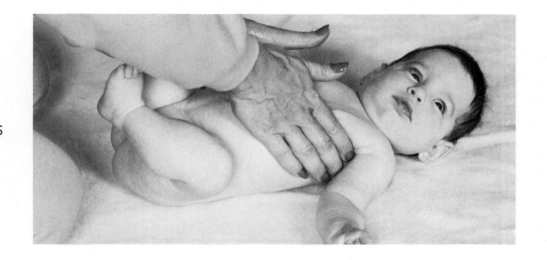

Arms and Hands

By massaging your baby's arms, you help stimulate circulation, which in turn stimulates muscle growth.

1.

Place your baby on his back and clasp his left hand in your left hand. Lift his arm up, placing your right hand under his left shoulder. Stroke your right hand down your baby's arm to clasp your baby's left hand.

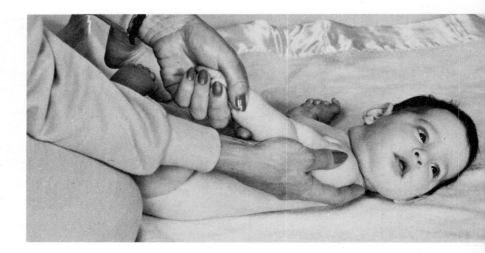

2.

Clasping your baby's left hand in your right hand, grasp his left arm underneath his shoulder and stroke downward with your left hand to clasp his hand. Repeat this sequence 6 times with both arms.

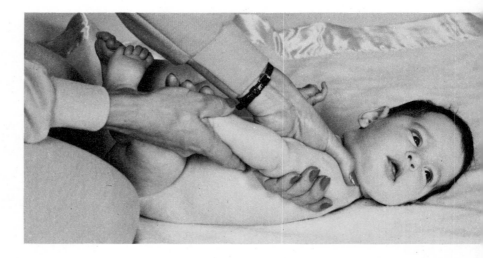

3.

Now hold your baby's left hand in your left hand while you clasp his left forearm with your right hand. Slide your right hand down his forearm, over and around his wrist, to grasp his left hand in your right.

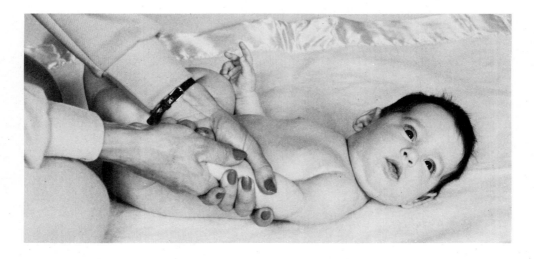

4.

Hold your baby's left forearm in your right hand and gently massage his left hand with your fingers. Repeat the sequence 6 times and change hands, repeating the sequence another 6 times.

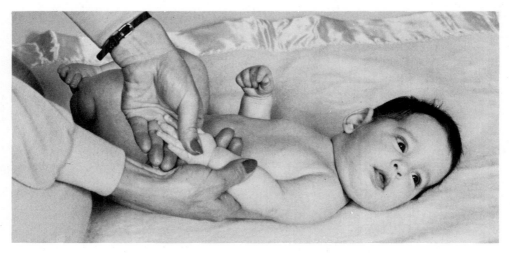

Hips and Bottom I

Not only are you stimulating circulation in this exercise, but the motion of your hands helps the muscles relax and function smoothly and

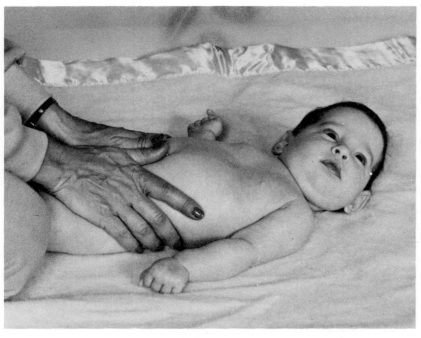

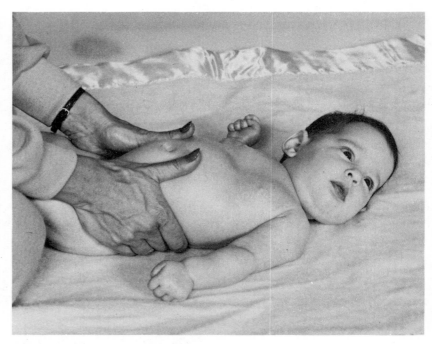

1. Place your baby on his back and put your hands on the front of his hips, above his thighs.

2. Stroke both hands outward until your fingers meet behind on your baby's lower back. You will probably be able to encircle your baby's entire waist.

properly. This in turn enables the internal organs to work properly.

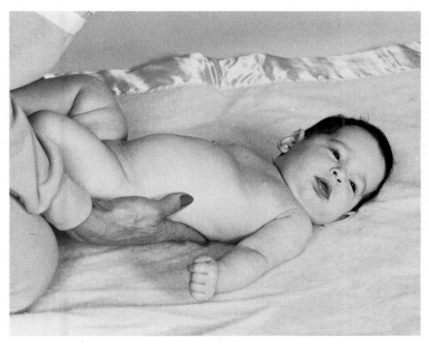

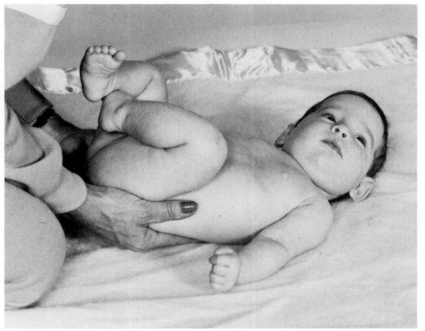

3. Reach your hands further around your baby's hips and massage his bottom and lower back area.

4. Lift your baby slightly off the quilt and stroke downward across his bottom and back around his hips so that your hands meet in their original position. Repeat the sequence 6 times.

Legs I

Stimulating the circulation in your baby's legs is important for proper muscle growth. By stretching and straightening the legs, you will also help

1.

Place your baby on his back and put your hands alongside his hips and thighs.

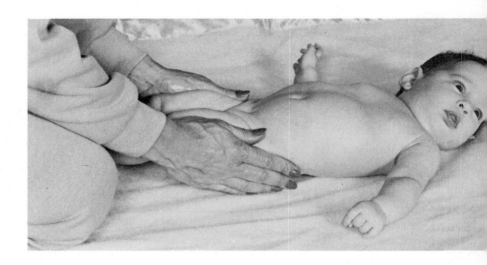

2.

Clasping your baby's legs in both of your hands, slowly stroke your hands downward over his thighs.

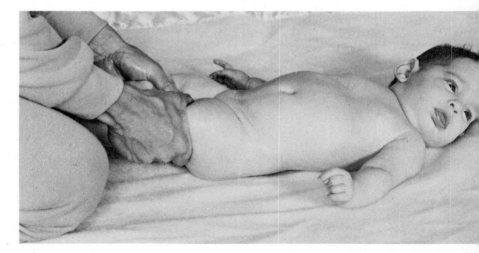

keep your baby's hamstring muscles flexible.

3.

Stroke down to your baby's ankles, still clasping his legs in your hands. Repeat the sequence 6 times.

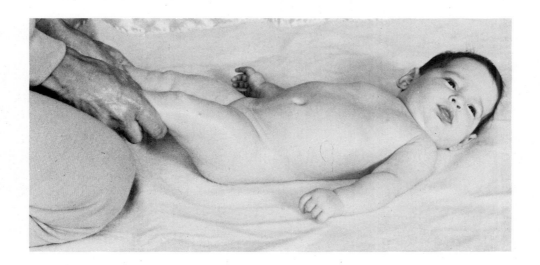

Legs and Feet

In addition to stimulating leg circulation and gently exercising hip muscles, this exercise benefits your baby's feet, which are the last areas of the body to receive

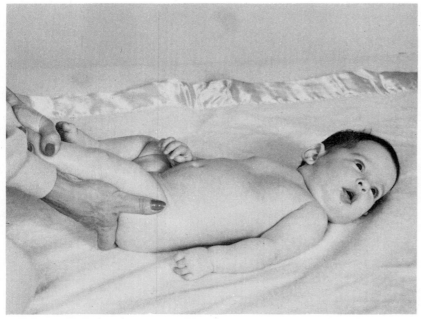

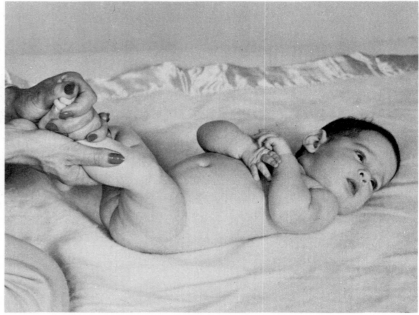

1. Place your baby on his back. As you clasp his left ankle in your left hand, place your right hand around the back and top part of his thigh, just below his bottom.

2. Stroke your right hand down your baby's entire leg to meet your left hand at his ankle. Then clasp his foot and stroke it from heel to toes, putting pressure on the sole of his foot with your thumb. Repeat 6 times.

blood and nutrition. By massaging them after you have massaged the legs, you ensure proper circulation and growth.

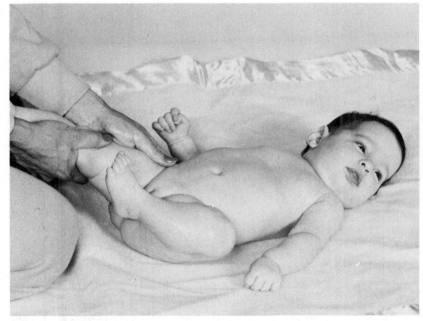

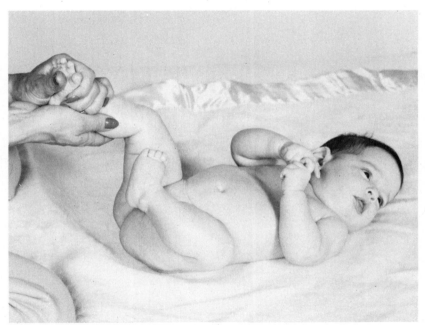

3. Now clasp your baby's right ankle in your right hand and place your left hand around the back and top part of his thigh, just below his bottom.

4. Stroke your left hand down your baby's entire leg to meet your right hand at his ankle. Clasp his foot and stroke it from heel to toes, putting pressure on the sole of his foot with your thumb. Repeat this sequence 6 times.

Back and Shoulders

By massaging your baby's back and shoulders, you can help relieve tension in that area. Babies sleep better when these muscles are relaxed.

1.

Place your baby on his tummy. Put your hands on his back with your fingertips toward his shoulders and the heels of your hands resting in the small of his back.

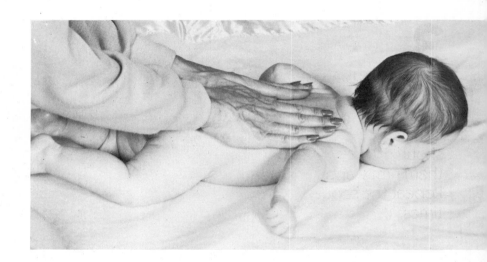

2.

Slowly stroke your hands upward over your baby's shoulders.

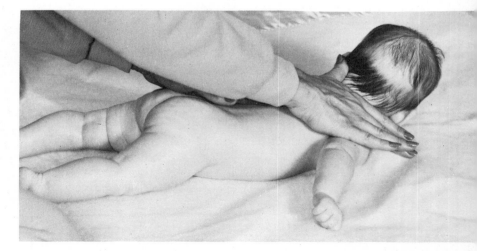

3.

Grasp your baby's shoulders and upper arms in your hands and continue to massage shoulders while gripping them firmly and gently. Repeat the sequence 6 times.

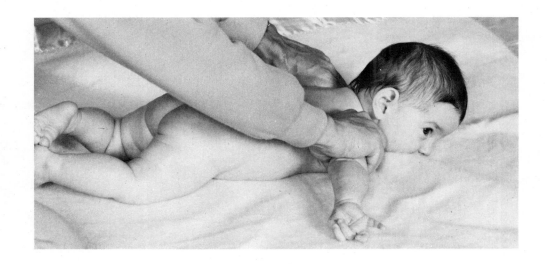

Hips and Bottom II

Massaging your baby's bottom and hips enables your child to feel motion in the pelvic area, the area that controls the entire torso. Your baby will

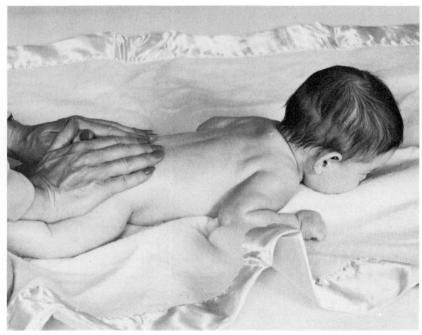

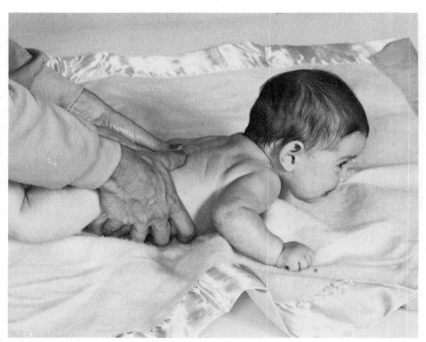

1. Place your baby on his tummy and cover his bottom with your hands. Your fingers should be resting on the small of his back and the heels of your hands should rest on his upper thighs.

2. Slowly stroke your hands up to the small of your baby's back, and reach your fingers around his waist while gently lifting your baby's hips up slightly.

tighten and relax muscles as you massage, which will increase their strength even before you start the regular exercise program.

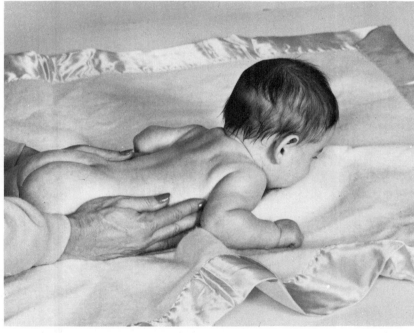

3. Bring your hands down alongside his waist, and stroke down his hips and thighs on both sides with the entire palm of your hand. Repeat the sequence 6 times.

Back and Bottom

Circulation is increased and back muscles are relaxed as you stimulate the muscles from just below the bottom to the shoulders.

1.

Place your baby on his tummy and clasp his right ankle with your right hand. Place your left hand on the right side of your baby's bottom.

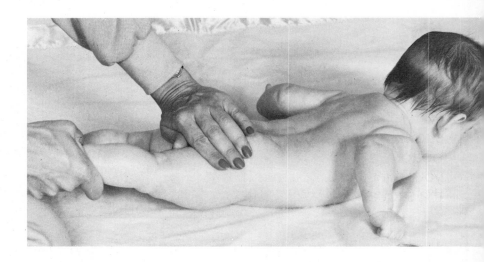

2.

Stroke your left hand up to your baby's right shoulder. Then grasp his right thigh and stroke downward until your left hand rests on the right side of his bottom.

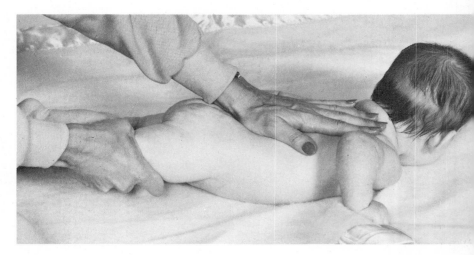

3.

In the same manner, clasp your baby's left leg with your left hand and stroke the left side of his bottom and back with your right hand. Repeat the sequence 6 times.

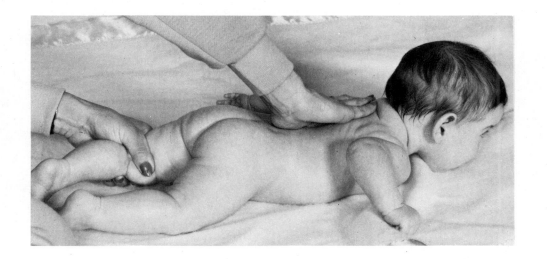

Legs II

Leg cramps are caused by poor circulation. By stimulating circulation and ensuring proper blood flow, chances of cramping are lessened.

1.

Place your baby on his tummy and hold his right foot in your right hand. Clasp his right thigh in your left hand and stroke downward to his ankle with your whole hand.

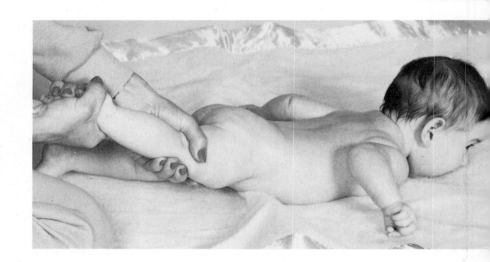

2.

Clasp your baby's right foot in your left hand and encircle his right thigh in your right hand. Stroke all the way down his ankle.

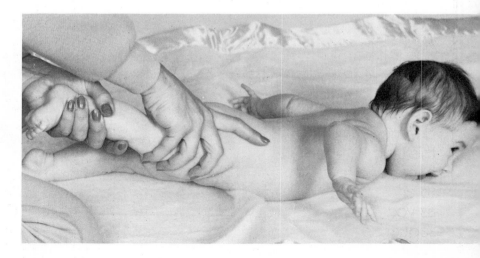

3.

Now clasp your baby's right foot in your right hand again, and stroke his right leg upward from the ankle to the thigh with your whole hand.

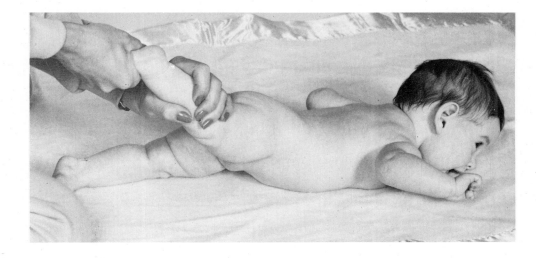

4.

Change legs and repeat the downward and upward stroking motions described in steps 1-3, this time with reverse hands and feet. Be sure to encircle the entire leg as you stroke. Repeat the sequence 6 times.

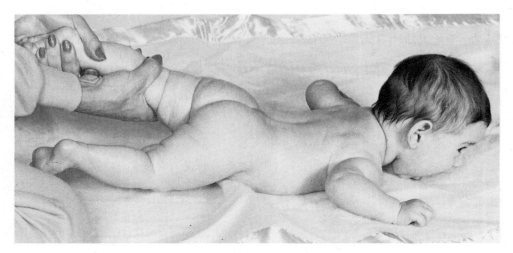

Rib Cage and Arms

This massage movement stimulates circulation in the chest, rib cage, arms, and armpits as it releases tension in the shoulders.

1.

Place your baby on his tummy and clasp his chest with both your hands so that he is slightly propped up. Then, while holding the right side of your baby's chest with your right hand, stroke outward along his left armpit and left arm with your left hand.

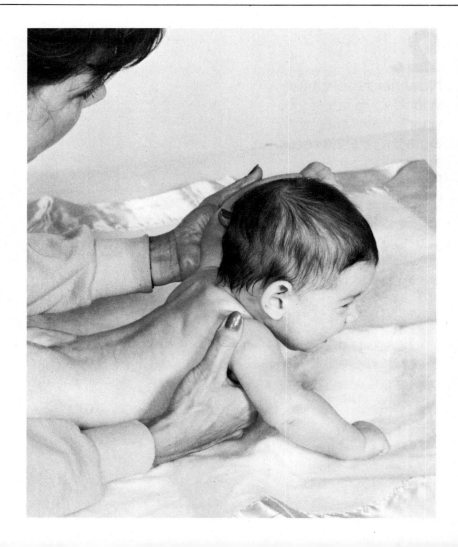

2.

Now hold the left side of your baby's chest with your left hand and stroke along his right armpit and arm with your right hand. Repeat the sequence 6 times.

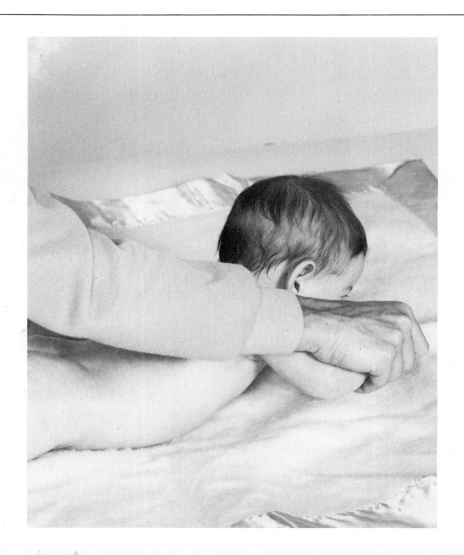

Infants: 4 Weeks to 3 Months

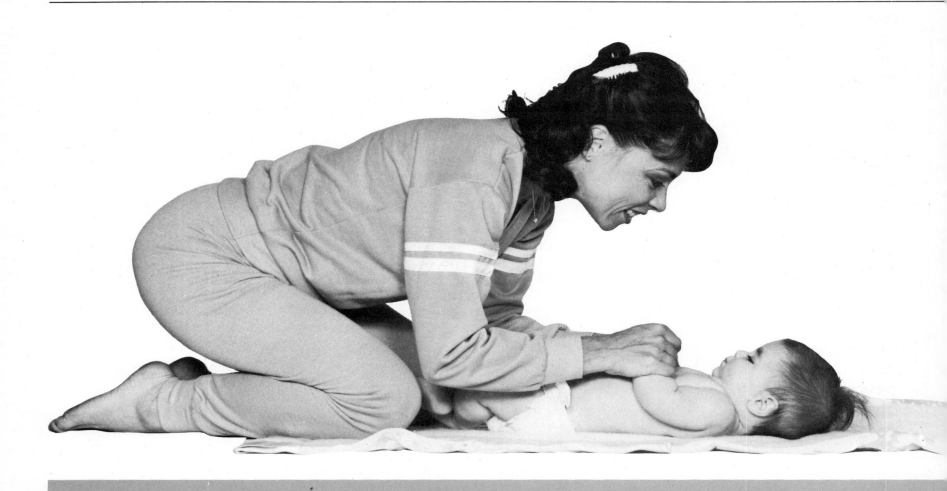

When babies are born, they have been curled up in the uterus for nine months. Then, all of a sudden, their muscles are asked to work properly, as if they had been stretched out all along. This is simply not possible. Place a baby on his back and he will automatically bend his knees and draw his arms forward. Place a baby on his side and he will curl up into the fetal position.

This is perfectly natural. But what does it mean in terms of muscle strength and weakness? Quite simply, the muscles in the chest (pectorals) are too tight and short, while the back and shoulder muscles are too long and stretched. Your baby will uncurl in the course of time. But exercise helps accelerate the process. By gently exercising your baby, you help strengthen his upper and lower back while stretching his chest and hip muscles.

The torso, especially the abdominal and lower back areas, controls the body. By making sure your infant's torso muscles work properly, you help ensure a lifetime of correct muscle function. By strengthening the upper back and stretching the pectorals, you help prevent future awkwardness and create proper muscle structure in your child, which will permit good posture later on.

The exercises in this section are designed to stimulate the whole body. What may look like an arm exercise only will also work the muscles in your baby's chest and upper back. The leg exercises will work the abdominals, lower back, and buttock muscles as well. The reason you shift from area to area is to avoid overworking any muscle group. As you shift back and forth, you rest a previously exercised area. Muscles should always be refreshed and energized after a workout—not sore or overworked.

Studies have shown that handling, cuddling, and hugging your baby is very beneficial for him, emotionally as well as physically. Each time a baby is picked up, he tightens the muscles in his body and then relaxes them as you hold him. Put another way, picking a baby up causes him to do isometric exercises. As with adults doing isometric exercise, the muscles are exercised slowly and then get progressively stronger. Although the baby doesn't seem to be "working" (you are doing all the pulling and pushing), each time you move a baby's limbs the muscles are actually stretching and releasing. During an entire arm movement of six seconds, a baby may tighten his muscles for a mere half second, an almost infinitesimal period of time.

But he is actually responding. His brain is registering the action, and his muscles are getting just a little bit stronger.

It is important to remember that babies tire very easily. A baby is constantly developing and growing, and that takes energy. Just being awake is a full-time activity for the infant. Babies more than double their weight in the first few months after birth. And not only are their muscles growing, their minds are becoming aware. Their senses are awakening. A baby is under a constant barrage of unfamiliar stimuli. Sight, sound, smell, heat, cold—all these things are new. The growth of the baby's senses, coupled with his actual physical growth, is difficult for us to comprehend and exhausting to the infant. This is the reason babies sleep so much. So remember: it's not just the exercises that are tiring your child; it's the entire growth process.

It is not possible to overstimulate a baby if you pay attention. When babies have had enough stimulation, they will let you know with a tired face or perhaps a whimper. If you watch and listen carefully, they will not even need to cry. You'll be able to tell when it's time to stop. If your child is fussy, try calming him with exercise. If he *becomes* fussy during exercise, stop.

The amount of time spent exercising is really up to your baby. You will probably shorten the time in the beginning. I suggest starting with five or ten minutes. Don't try to do every exercise in one session. But if you add a few new ones every so often, you will soon find that you are finishing the whole program quite happily and comfortably in one day. It is a good idea to massage your baby first, then exercise, then massage again.

As with massage, it doesn't matter what time of day you exercise your baby. Your baby should be alert and comfortable. All you need is a soft quilt and some pleasant music. I always recommend using music when exercising your child. Keeping time to music is not only enjoyable, it helps communicate rhythm and coordination. And exercise seems easier and more pleasant when it is accompanied by music.

Place your baby on a quilt on the floor. He should be naked whenever possible. Put the music on and begin. When you are finished exercising your baby, massage him briefly and then hug him.

In the beginning your baby will allow you to do all the work. But remember that although he's passive at this time, his muscles are being used and therefore worked. Later, he will begin to work with you or against you. Don't worry if he occasionally doesn't want to exercise at all. If you make today's session as pleasant as possible, he will be inclined to want to repeat the process tomorrow.

Thumb Grip

Practice the Thumb Grip often with your infant. It builds strength in his hands, and is used in many of these early exercises.

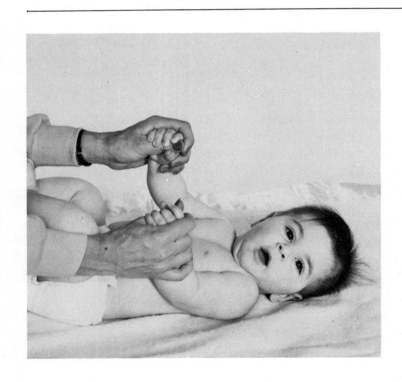

Place your baby on his back and have him clasp your thumbs in his hands. Place your fingers over his hands to secure his grip. As your baby's exercise program progresses, you will find that his grip on your thumbs becomes tighter and more sure as his hands become stronger. Your grasp can relax somewhat. Eventually he will hold your thumbs without your holding on to his hands at all.

Arm Cross

While focusing attention on your baby's arms during this exercise, the pectoral and upper back muscles are also being stretched and strengthened.

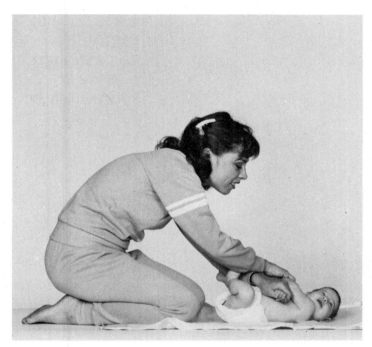

1. Place your baby on his back and have him clasp your hands in the thumb grip. Cross your baby's arms across his chest.

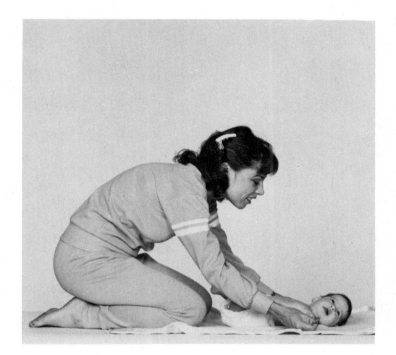

2. Stretch your baby's arms straight out to his sides at shoulder height. Repeat the sequence 8 times.

Arm Raises

It is important for your baby to have flexible shoulders. This simple routine exercises shoulders while it stretches your baby's arm muscles.

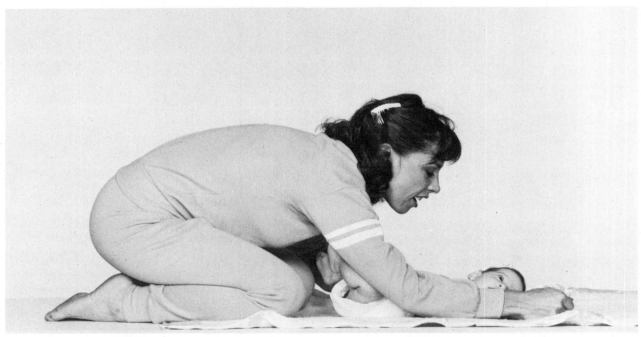

1. Place your baby on his back and have him grasp your hands in the thumb grip. Raise your baby's arms straight above his head.

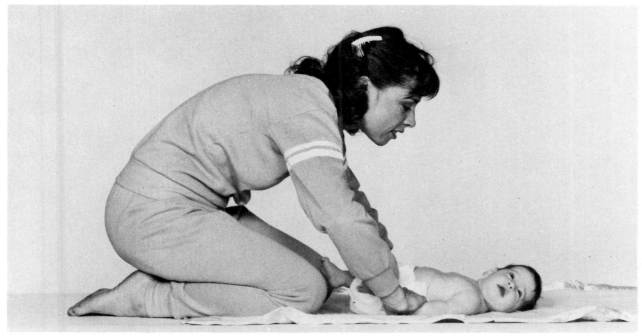

2. Lower your baby's arms to his sides. Repeat the sequence 8 times.

Alternate Arm Raises

Another shoulder exercise that also strengthens arms, pectorals, and upper back muscles. You can combine this exercise with the previous one.

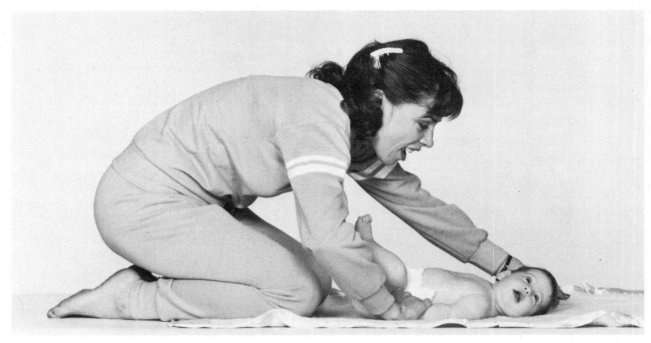

1. Place your baby on his back and have him grasp your hands in the thumb grip. Raise your baby's right arm straight over his head as you lower his straight left arm to his side.

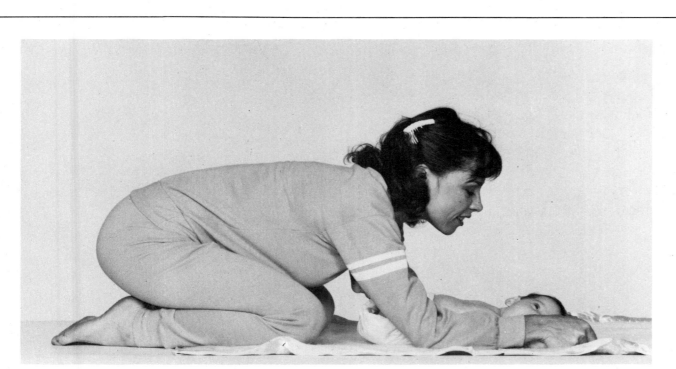

2. Slowly lower your baby's right arm as you raise his straight left arm over his head. Repeat the sequence 8 times.

Knee Bends

This basic exercise helps strengthen your baby's legs while enhancing hamstring flexibility. Be sure to straighten his legs completely after bending his knees.

1.

Place your baby on his back and clasp his legs in your hands. Hold them straight. Your thumbs should be resting on his shins while your fingers grasp his calf muscles.

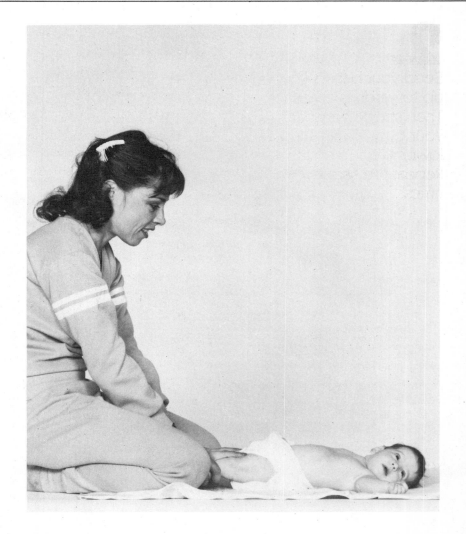

2.

Bend your baby's knees up toward his chest. Then straighten both of your baby's legs and lower them to the floor. Repeat the sequence 8 times.

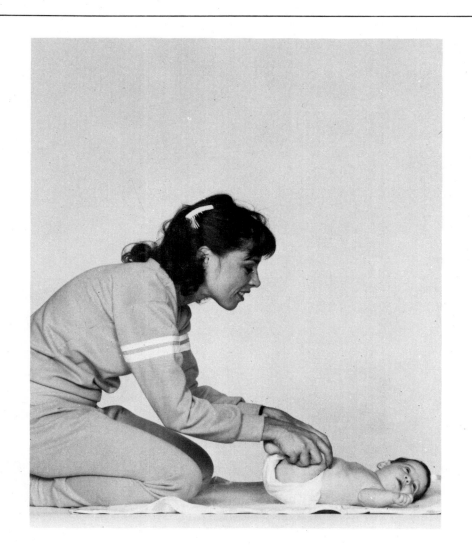

Alternate Knee Bends

This is excellent for leg strength and flexibility. Many mothers have found that this exercise relieves crankiness in their babies.

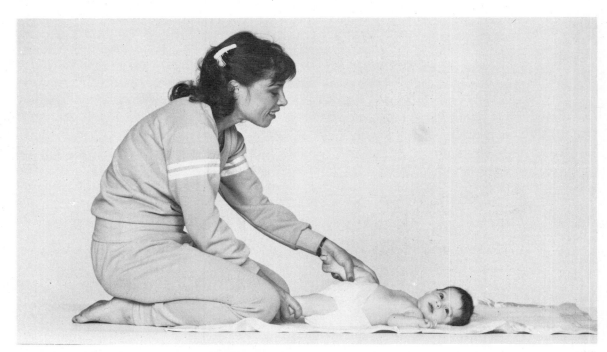

1. Place your baby on his back and clasp his calves in your hands. Bend your baby's right leg to push his right knee up to his chest while you straighten his left leg.

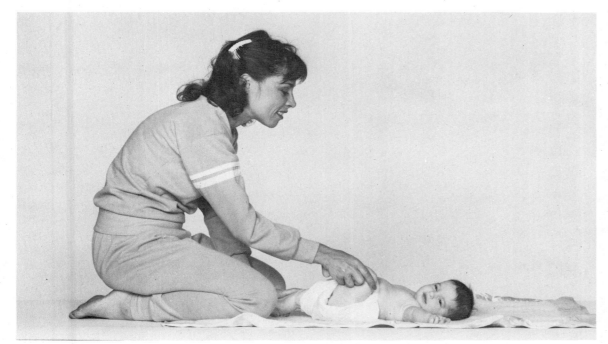

2. In a smooth and continuous motion, bend your baby's left knee up to his chest while you straighten and lower his right leg to the floor. Repeat the sequence 8 times.

Foot Flex

This exercise is especially good for your baby if his feet turn in or out. If they turn in, do extra turning-out repetitions. If they turn out, do extra turning-in

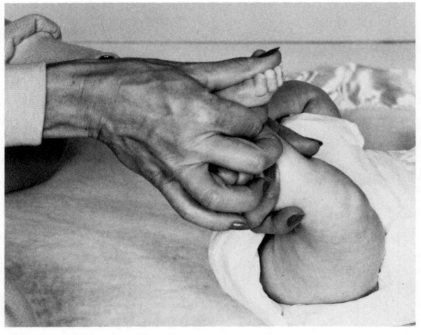

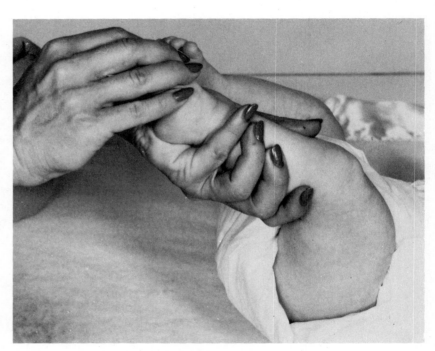

1. Place your baby on his back and clasp his left ankle in your left hand. With your right thumb on the ball of your baby's foot, press his foot upward into a flexed position.

2. With the fingers of your right hand above and your thumb under his toes, gently press your baby's foot downward into a pointed position. Repeat this sequence 6 times with each foot.

repetitions. Be sure that your baby's legs are held still and that only his feet move. Always wiggle each foot to relax it when you have finished doing this exercise.

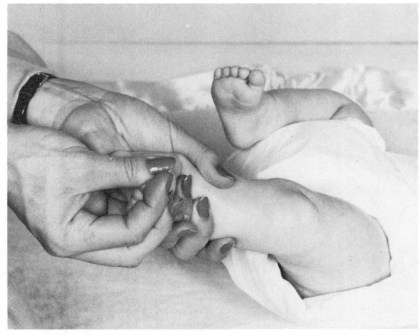

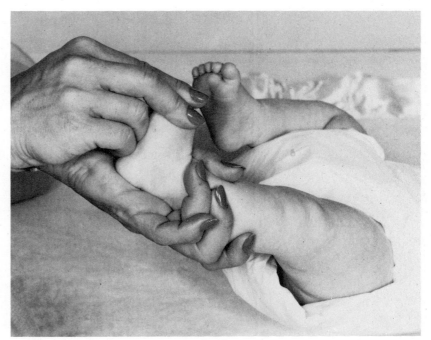

3. Grasp your baby's left ankle in your left hand, with your thumb resting on the instep of his foot. Gently turn his foot outward. Be sure to hold his ankle so that only his foot is moving.

4. Now turn your baby's foot inward, making sure his ankle is kept still so that only his foot is moving. Repeat this sequence 6 times with each foot.

Early Sit-Up

The abdominal muscles are the center point of the body, and therefore basically control the entire torso. This exercise helps strengthen these

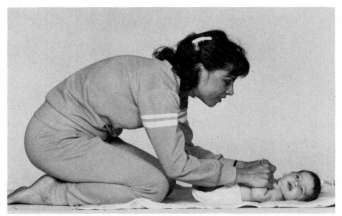

1.

Place your baby on his back and have him grasp your hands in the thumb grip.

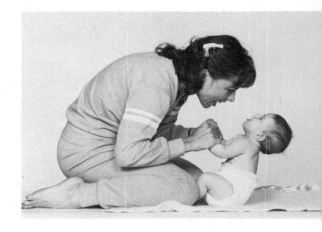

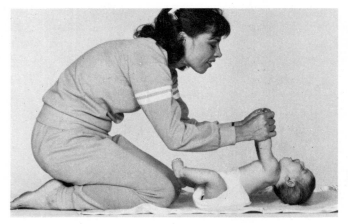

2.

Holding your baby's hands firmly, slowly and gently pull him up into a sitting position.

3.

Hold your baby in a sitting position for a few seconds.

important muscles. Your baby will allow you to do most of the work when you start doing this exercise, but as he gets stronger, he will begin to pull himself up.

Until your baby is strong enough to hold his head up by himself, you must support his head and neck when lowering him to the supine position.

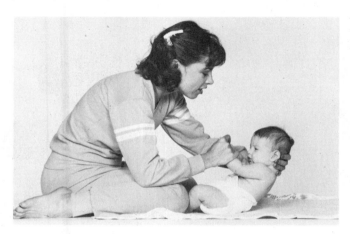

4.
Take both of your baby's hands in one of yours and place your free hand behind your baby's head and neck for support.

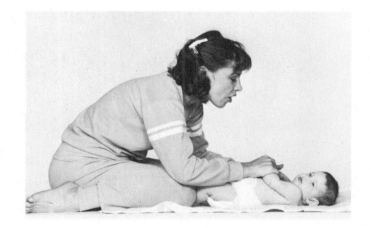

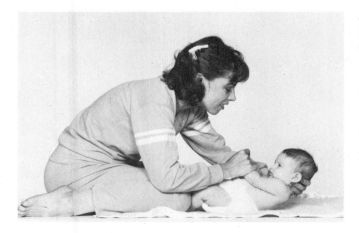

5.
Slowly lower your baby to a supine position with his back resting on the floor.

6.
Have your baby grasp both your hands in the thumb grip again. Repeat the sequence 4 times.

The Scooter

"**S**cooting" is a natural reflex action. If you put your hands against the soles of your baby's feet, he will automatically push against them while

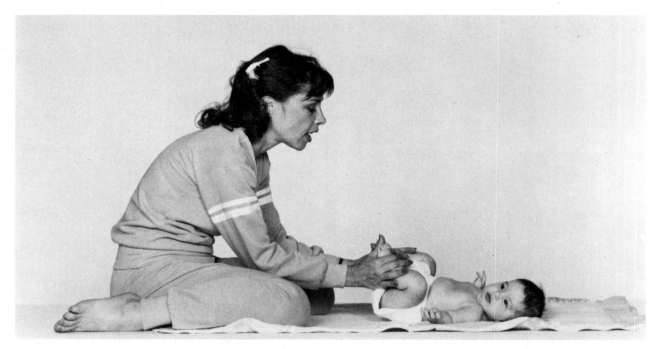

1. Place your baby on his back and clasp his feet and ankles. Bend his knees gently toward, but not over, his chest.

straightening his legs. By adding a little resistance, your baby will strengthen his leg muscles. In the beginning, your baby may kick his legs straight up in the air as shown here, but eventually he will straighten his legs so they are parallel to the floor.

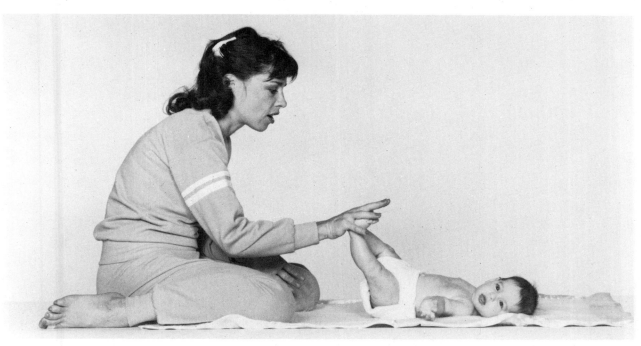

2. With your hands on the soles of your baby's feet, allow him to kick outward. Repeat the sequence 8 times.

Chest Lift

A strong upper back is necessary to hold the body straight. This exercise will help to strengthen your baby's upper back and shoulders. At the same

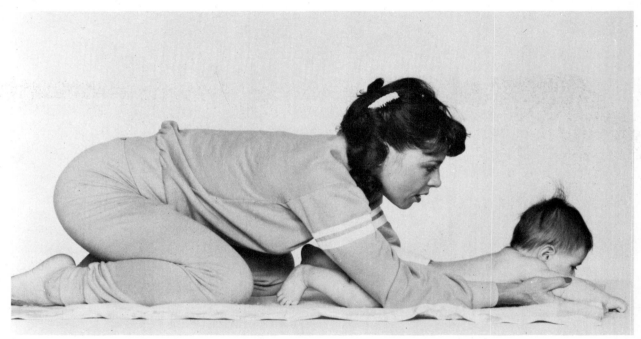

1. Place your baby on his tummy and grasp him under his arms with your fingers on his arms and the palms of your hands under his armpits.

time, you will be teaching him to lift his head and chest off the floor.

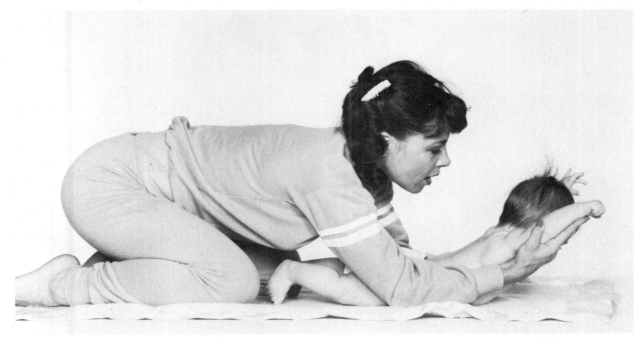

2. Slowly lift your baby's entire upper torso off the floor, making sure his tummy remains on the floor. Then lower his chest to the floor. Repeat the sequence 6 times.

Leg Lifts

This exercise helps strengthen your baby's lower back and ensure its flexibility as he becomes more active. Be sure his torso remains on the floor.

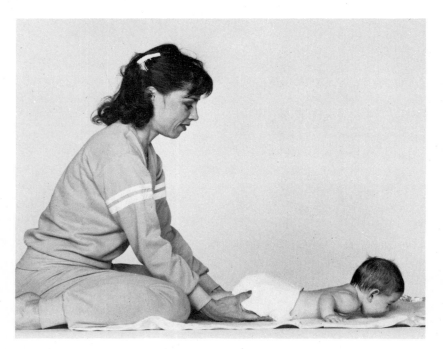

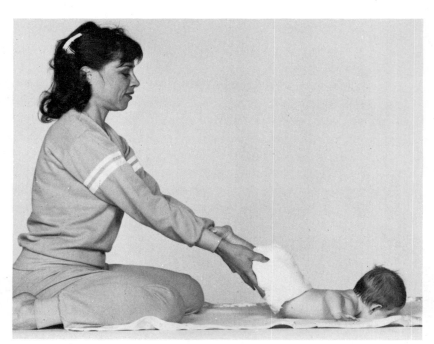

1. Place your baby on his tummy and grasp his thighs in your hands. Your thumbs should be on the back of his thighs while your fingers rest on the front of his upper thighs and on his hips.

2. Slowly and gently lift your baby's legs straight up so that his lower back is comfortably arched. Then lower your baby's straight legs to the floor. Repeat 6 times.

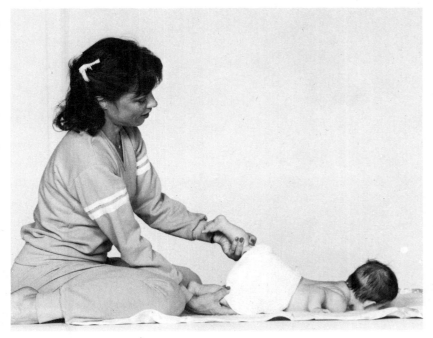

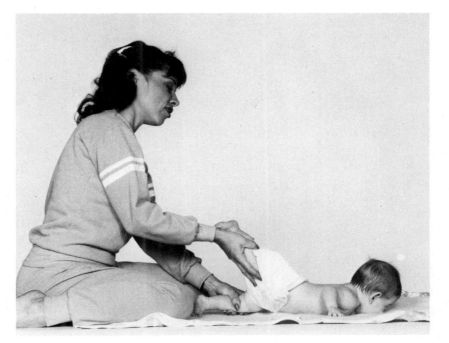

3. In a similar manner, lift your baby's left leg, keeping his right leg on the floor.

4. Lower your baby's left leg while you lift his right leg. Repeat this sequence 6 times.

Frog Kick

No one expects an infant to crawl at one, two, or three months, but this exercise helps strengthen his legs so that crawling is easier when the time is right.

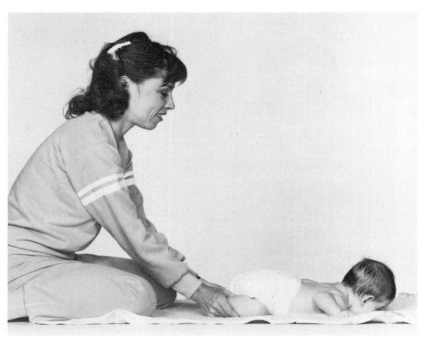

1. Place your baby on his tummy and grasp his calves in your hands. Keeping his legs on the floor, slowly bend his knees to the side while gently pushing his feet up toward his crotch.

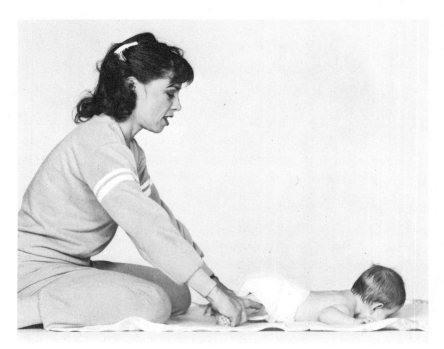

2. Straighten and spread your baby's legs out to the sides. Do not pull hard on his legs.

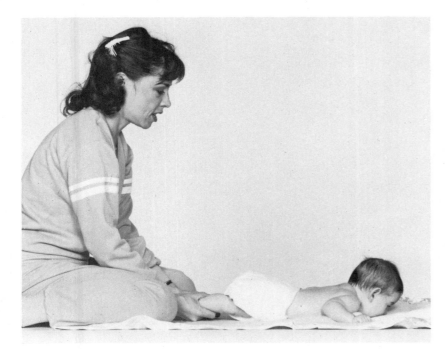

3. Bring your baby's legs together, keeping them straight, with his knees facing the floor. Repeat the sequence 8 times.

Infants:
4 to 11 Months

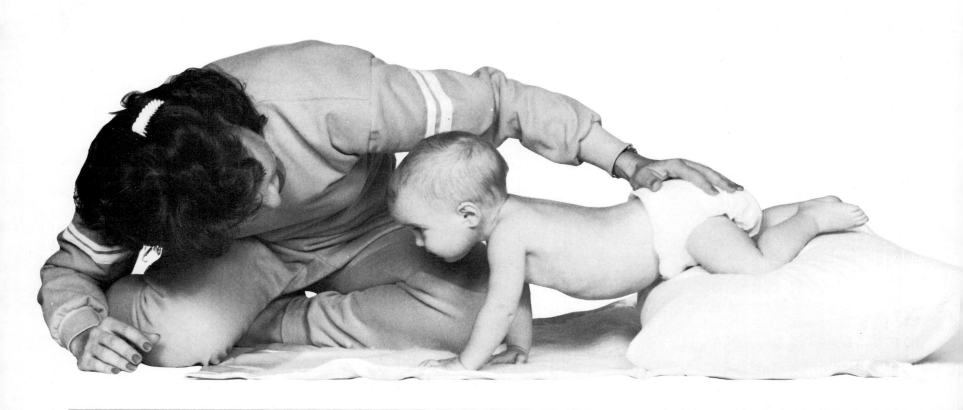

At four months, your child is more alert during his waking hours than he was at three months. Those periods of time when your baby is awake should be intense learning sessions. Talking to your child is very important, because it helps him begin to understand language. For that matter, everything you do with and for your baby is being stored in your child's brain for future use.

Your child will definitely respond to many different forms of stimulation at this point. He may kick and squirm happily when he sees your face, whereas before he may have looked at you passively. Your child is aware. He is showing you that he is noticing what is going on.

He is also beginning to know that every action generates a reaction. If he cries, he knows you will come to his aid. If he does something, you will respond. Now is the time he begins to develop his self-esteem. If he does something to cause you to react with pleasure, he feels good about himself–and will probably want to do it again.

You will see definite changes in your child when you exercise him. Before, your child passively allowed you to manipulate his limbs. Now, the Bicycle exercise will often elicit a contented smile.

You can feel your baby's strength now, too. It starts with a slight resistance while exercising, a grabbing at things and not letting go. He has also begun to hold and push for longer periods of time. At times he may resist so much that you have to stop for a moment. He is not being negative here; if he didn't want to exercise, he would cry. He is working his muscles. If he tries to keep his arm bent when you want to straighten it, he is helping you to help him become stronger.

If this becomes a battle and you have difficulty moving his limbs at all because he resists so much, change exercises. You don't want to fight the muscles, you just want some give and take. There will be days when your child may seem very pliant and others when he is totally resistant. I hope that most days will begin to fall somewhere in between.

Now is the time when strengthening the upper back and stretching the chest are extremely important. Your baby will be sitting soon, and you want to be sure that he has proper posture. The Sit-Up with Dowel is a good exercise, as is the Early Push-Up. The sit-up strengthens mainly the abdominals, which help hold the sitting position. The push-up stretches and strengthens the pectorals and the upper back muscles, enabling your baby to hold the sitting position correctly.

Crawling is just around the corner. You want your baby to experience as little frustration as possible when he is learning to crawl. Doing the Crawl Push exercise gives baby an idea of where his legs should be placed when crawling. You are not teaching your baby to crawl sooner than he normally would, you are strengthening his muscles so that he will know how to maneuver his body when he starts to crawl.

As you exercise your child, you are helping him develop his entire musculature. Abdominal muscles are becoming stronger for sitting, back and chest muscles are being strengthened for proper posture, and legs are developing for crawling and eventually walking. Your baby's arms can now support his chest and, when he holds something, you may notice he has quite a grip. His hands are becoming stronger with the help of the Thumb Grip exercise you've been doing.

You will also notice that your baby is developing definite eye-hand coordination. This means that your child is learning to coordinate vision with movement. He will no longer just gesture at an object, but, as he focuses on it, he will begin to reach directly for it. He is becoming smoother, more systematic and selective in his movements.

During this period, your baby will become more skillful in everything he does. He not only simply enjoys doing things for his own sake, but also because something else happens as a result of his movement. Clapping hands makes a noise, kicking a blanket makes it fall off, putting a hand over his eye makes it dark on one side. These are games that increase a child's intelligence and awareness as well as his motor control.

Dr. Willibald Nagler, Chief of Rehabilitation Medicine for the N.Y. Hospital-Cornell Medical Center, says: "The baby doesn't kick a ball for a specific purpose; the kicking itself gives pleasure." So too with obstacles such as the pillow. Watch your child struggle through this exercise and then experience the joy of his having accomplished it.

This is a time of rapid development in your child, both physically and intellectually. But it is important to remember that each baby grows at his own pace. Age is not important here. What is important is that your baby is happy and healthy and that you notice a continuing process of forward development. As long as you are working with your child and helping him to become strong and well-coordinated, he will reach each plateau on time. *His* time. It is a time for discovery. Your child is becoming aware of the world outside of him. He is still concerned with his own needs, but now he knows how to get what he wants instead of just waiting for it to be handed to him.

Try setting obstacles in front of a baby of eight months to keep him from getting to an object he wants. He will move anything he can (small stools, a chair, empty boxes) out of the way so that he can reach his destination. If you watch a baby when he is alone, you will see the seeds of logic developing in him. Offer these seeds the proper nutrition (that is, continue to put your child in situations where he must, and easily can, use thought and then body to get what he wants), and logic as well as coordination will blossom.

I have included the use of a dowel and a pillow in this section. Be aware, though, that babies at this age are often ready to use more advanced forms of equipment. Although exercises are not shown in this section for use with a ladder or a ramp, many babies, as stated in the introduction, love to climb up or across them as soon as they are able. I start babies on this equipment at my school as soon as they can crawl, so

use your own discretion here. Start introducing additional equipment as soon as you feel you both are ready. Use the articles mentioned above (included in this and the next section) and also make up uses for other items you may have around the house.

You may do the basic exercises on a quilt, but you will find your baby scooting off of it as soon as he is able. Of course, the floor is the safest place to exercise. Your child will visibly respond to the beat of music now, so use it. Choose music that is happy and makes you feel good.

The time of day you exercise is up to you. At four to six months, you will find your baby can be exercised for longer than five to ten minutes. You can easily go from fifteen minutes up to half an hour, but I recommend cutting the session slightly shorter than you have to so that your baby finishes while he is in a happy mood. This keeps the memory of each session pleasant. As he gets older, your baby can work out for well over half an hour. But *always* stop if he becomes fussy and cranky. Remember that each day is different. When you finish, it is always nice to massage and hug your child.

Leg Cross

It is extremely important for babies to have flexible torsos. This exercise strengthens your baby's torso muscles and eventually helps him learn to turn

1.

Place your baby on his back and clasp his calves in your hands.

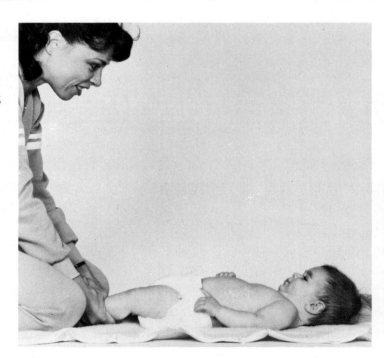
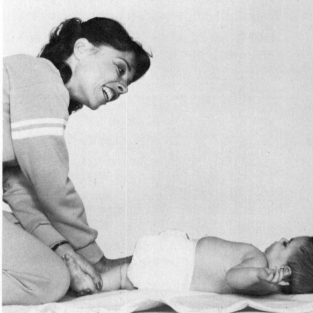

over by himself. It also stretches the leg
and hip muscles.

2.

Raise your baby's left leg
off the floor and cross it
over his right leg, placing
the foot on the floor and
allowing his knee to
bend slightly. The left
side of his torso should
twist upward so that his
hip is raised toward the
ceiling.

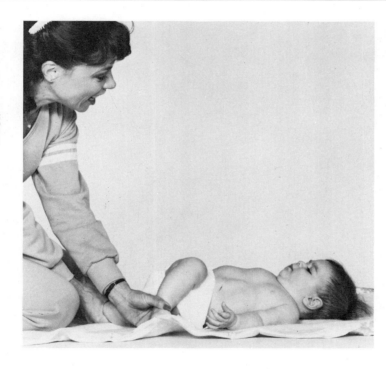

3.

Return your baby's left
leg to the floor and raise
his right leg up to cross
over the left in the same
manner. Repeat the
sequence 8 times.

The Bicycle

Both your baby's abdominal muscles and his legs get a good workout with this exercise. Be sure to keep the circular movements smooth and even.

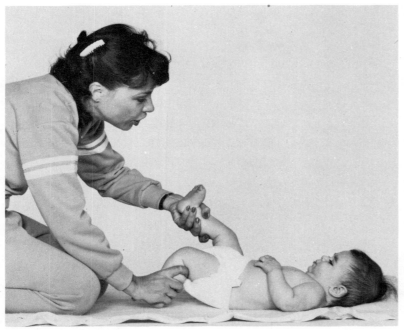

1. Place your baby on his back and clasp his calves in your hands. Raise his right leg up and forward.

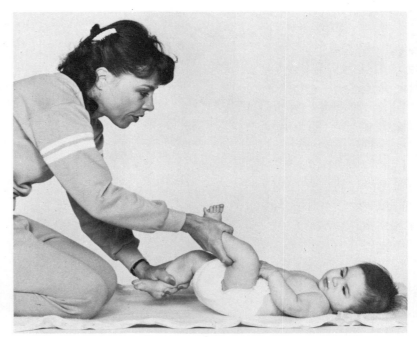

2. Slowly rotate his legs in a forward circular motion, raising the left leg up and forward while lowering the right leg down and back, as if your baby were riding a bicycle. Complete 16 rotations.

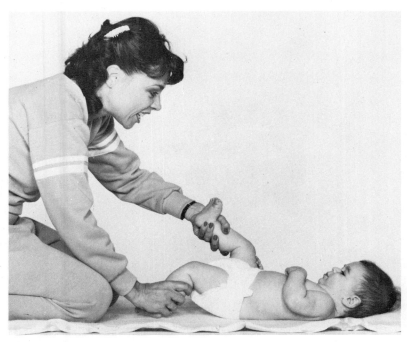

3. Then change direction and rotate his left leg backward and down while you bring his right leg forward and up.

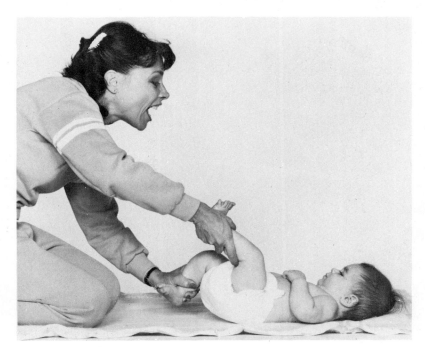

4. Rotate the legs in a backward bicycle motion to complete 16 rotations.

Knee Bend and Arm Stretch

A favorite of most babies, this exercise uses the full stretch of your baby's arms and legs. It is excellent for coordination and flexibility.

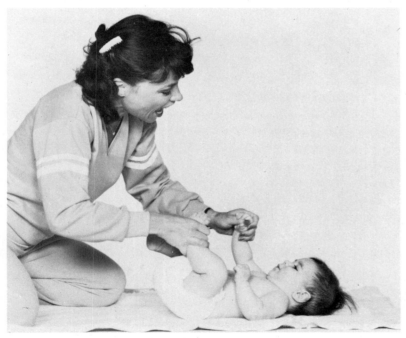

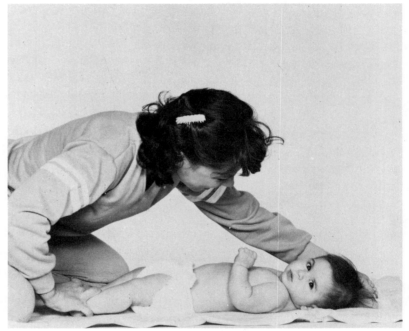

1. Place your baby on his back. Have him grasp your left hand with his right while you hold his left calf in your right hand. Bring your baby's left foot up and his right hand down so that they meet.

2. Now stretch his right arm straight over your baby's head as you straighten and stretch his left leg down to the floor.

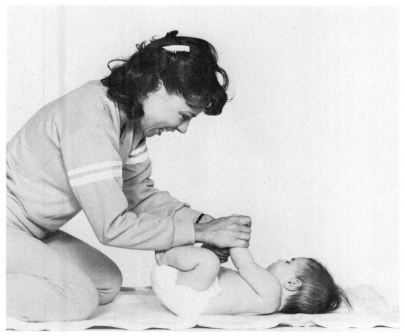

3. Change hands, and in the same manner bring your baby's right foot up to meet his left hand over his torso.

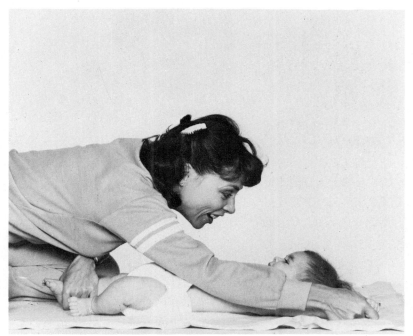

4. Then stretch his left arm straight over his head as you straighten and stretch his right leg. Repeat the sequence 10 times.

Toes-to-Nose

Babies adore this exercise. Not only does it produce much laughter, but it strengthens abdominal and lower back muscles and stretches leg muscles.

1.

Place your baby on his back and clasp both calves in your hands. Your thumbs should rest on his calf muscles while your fingers cover his shins. Bring your baby's right foot up to touch his nose, allowing his left leg to come off the floor.

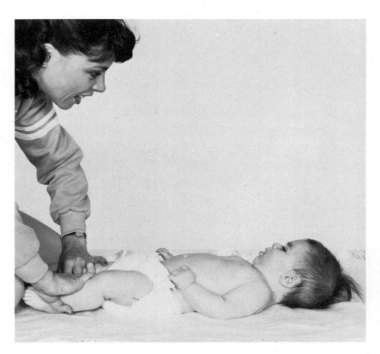
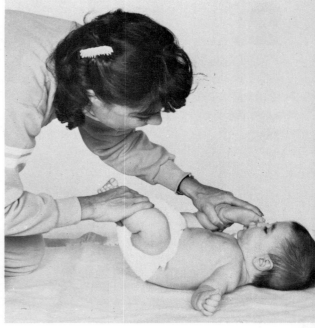

2.

Straighten your baby's right leg and bring both legs down to the floor with his knees toward the ceiling.

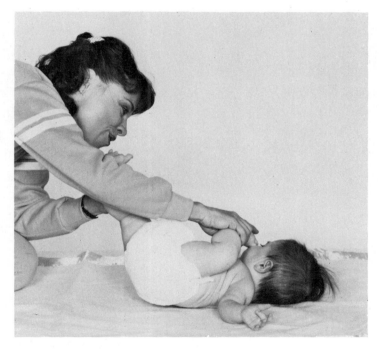

3.

Bring your baby's left foot up to touch his nose, allowing his right leg to come off the floor. Straighten both legs and bring them to the floor. Repeat the sequence 8 times.

Overhead Leg Stretch

In this exercise, the lower back and abdominal muscles are strengthened while the hamstring muscles are stretched and made more flexible. Raise

1.

Place your baby on his back and raise his legs, clasping them in your hands with your thumbs on the back of his legs and your fingers covering his knees.

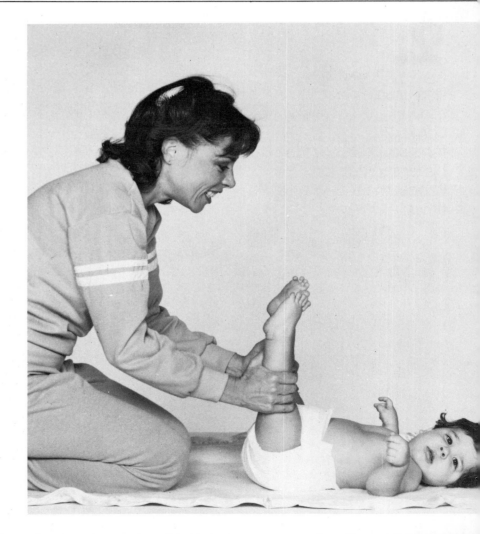

your baby's legs up and over his head only as far as he can comfortably go. Don't force. Each week he will be able to stretch his legs a little more, eventually reaching over his head.

2.

Slowly lift your baby's legs up over his torso, allowing his bottom to come off the floor. Hold for 2 seconds, then lower his legs to the floor. Repeat the sequence 8 times.

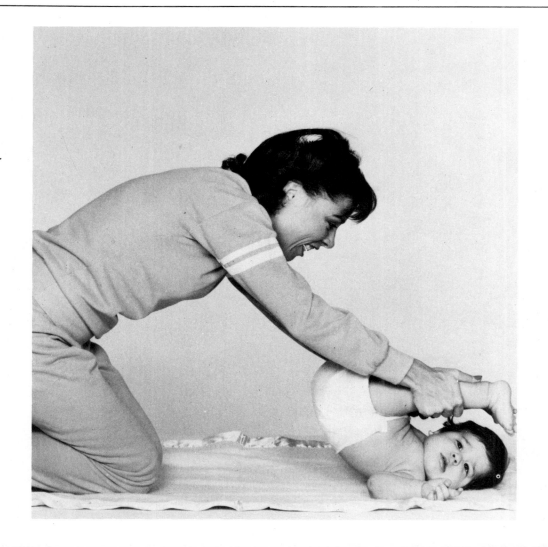

The Hang

This exercise may seem a little frightening to you at first, but it is extremely enjoyable for your child and is excellent for arm, back, chest, and

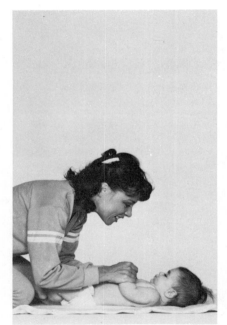

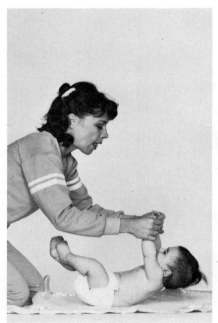

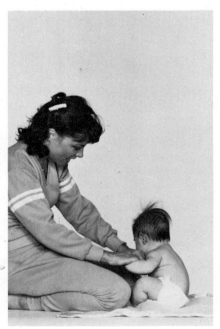

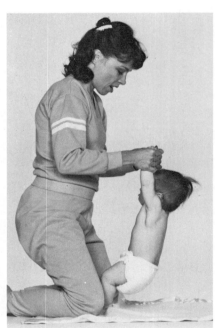

1.
Place your baby on his back and have him grasp your hands in the thumb grip.

2.
Slowly pull your baby up into a sitting position.

3.
Allow your baby to sit for a few seconds.

4.
Gently raise your baby's arms over his head and pull him upward.

shoulder strength. In the beginning, hold your baby in the air for only 3 seconds so that he does not strain his shoulders. As he becomes stronger, you will be able to hold him in the air for longer periods.

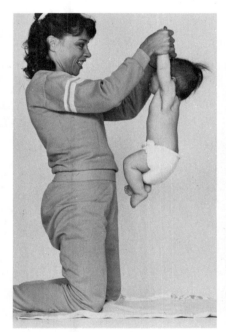

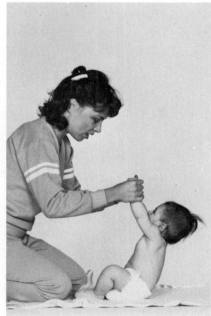

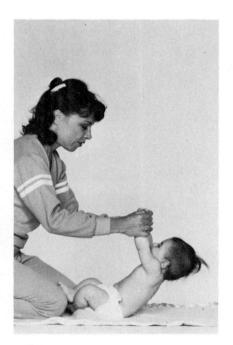

5.

Raise your baby off the floor and hold him in the air for 3 seconds.

6.

Slowly lower your baby to the floor.

7.

Lower your baby onto his back to the full supine position. Repeat the sequence 4 times, resting after each sequence.

Back Crossover

This exercise increases flexibility in the torso and legs while strengthening your baby's lower back. It also helps your baby learn how to use the muscles he

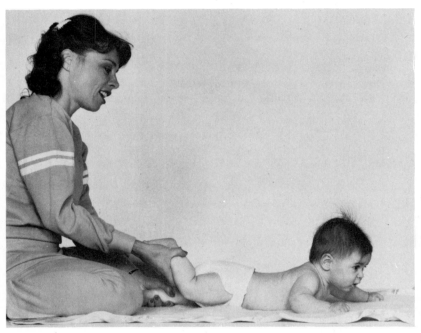

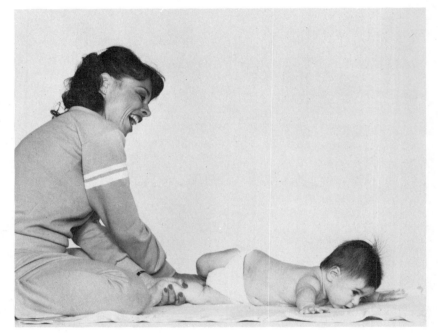

1. Place your baby on his tummy and clasp his calves in your hands. Your thumbs should rest behind his ankles and your fingers on his shins.

2. While holding your baby's left leg in place, lift his right leg up and cross it over and behind his left leg, placing the right foot on the floor. Allow his right hip to rise up toward the ceiling.

will need for turning himself over. Make sure you keep the movements smooth during this exercise.

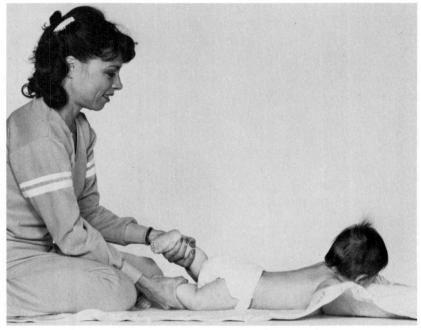

3. Lower his right leg to its original position and hold it there as your lift his left leg up and cross it over his right leg.

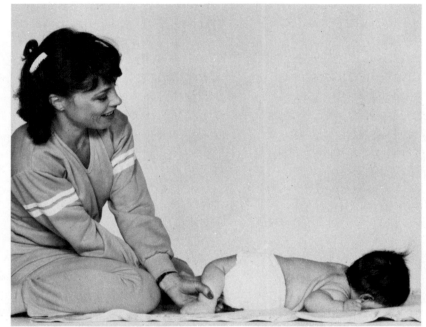

4. Place your baby's left foot on the floor, allowing his left hip to rise up toward the ceiling. Lower his left leg to its original position. Repeat the sequence 8 times.

The Crawl Push

Babies who do this exercise won't necessarily crawl sooner, but they will crawl with more dexterity. It is excellent for helping your baby learn

1.

Place your baby on his tummy and clasp his calves in your hands. Bend your baby's legs and push his knees out to the sides like a little frog's.

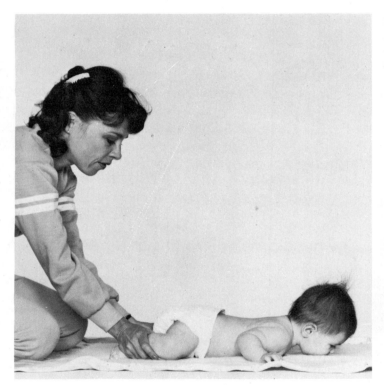
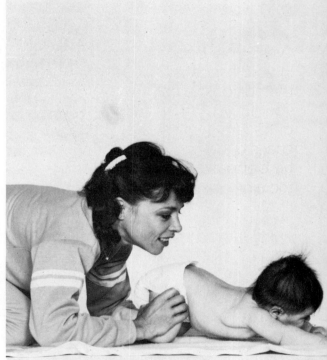

how to place his legs when crawling, and increases strength in the adductor (inner thigh) muscles.

2.◆

Grasp your baby's thighs in your hands with your thumbs on the back and your fingers on the front of his legs. Now slide his knees under him so that his bottom sticks up into the air.

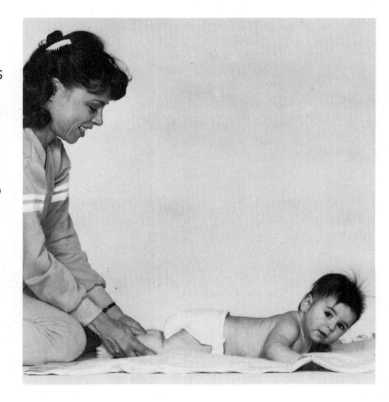

3.◆

Grasp your baby's calves again and pull his legs down so that his knees face downward and his legs are straight. Repeat the sequence 8 times.

Early Push-Up

Baby push-ups are excellent for strengthening arm, back, and pectoral muscles. It may take several attempts, however, before your baby knows to

1.

Place your baby on his tummy and clasp his upper thighs and hips. Have your baby support his torso on his hands.

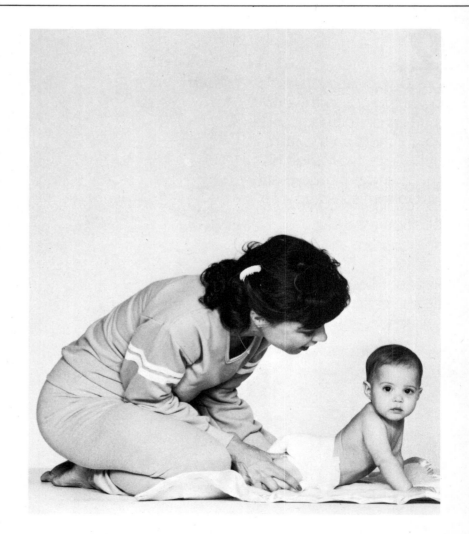

push up with his arms. Support his hips and tummy when you first start doing this exercise. As your baby gets older and stronger, you will be able to hold just his thighs, but be sure his back does not sag, as this indicates weakness and strain. If it does, go back to supporting his tummy and hips until he is stronger.

2.◆

Make sure your baby keeps his arms straight as you lift his hips off the floor no higher than the height of his arms, supporting his tummy as you lift. Hold this position for 4 seconds and then lower your baby's legs to the floor. Repeat the sequence 6 times, resting after each sequence.

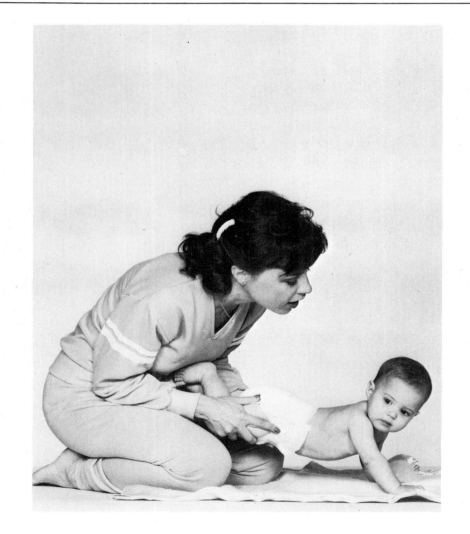

Upside-Down Hang

At first, some babies may be afraid to hang upside down. Don't force your child. However, the more you attempt this, the less frightened your child will be

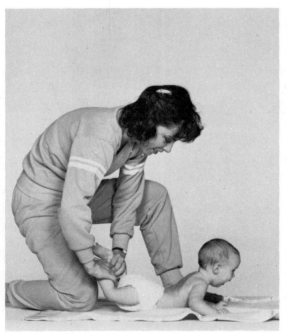

1.

Place your baby on his tummy and clasp his calves in your hands, with your thumbs on his shins and your fingers on his calf muscles.

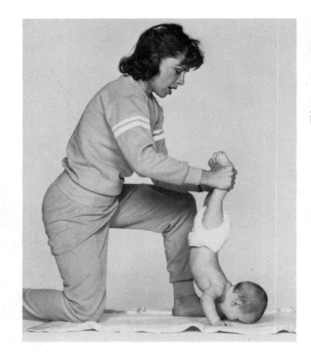

2.

Slowly lift your baby so that he is upside-down.

and it will soon become a preferred exercise. The Upside-Down Hang is excellent for strengthening arm, shoulder, chest, and back muscles as well as for stimulating circulation. It is also good for teaching babies how to protect their faces if they fall. Always do this exercise slowly.

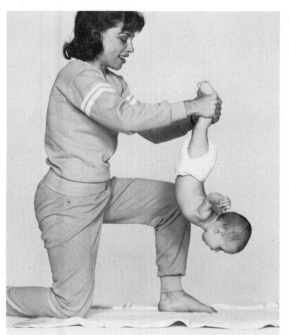

3.

Hold your baby in this upside-down position for 3 seconds, then slowly lower him to the floor.

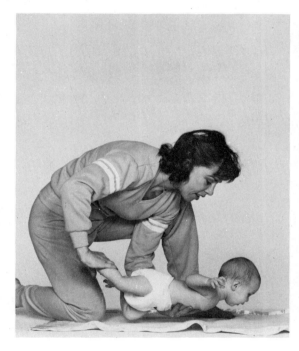

4.

Until your baby has learned to place his hands on the floor, help guide him by holding both feet in one hand while supporting his chest with the other. Allow him to rest. Repeat the sequence 4 times.

Arm Raises with Dowel

Babies love to hold on to things. With the help of this simple exercise, your baby will be able to strengthen his overall grip. Stretching his arms in this manner

1.

Place your baby on his back and have him grasp a dowel with both hands. Cover his hands with your fingers to secure his grip.

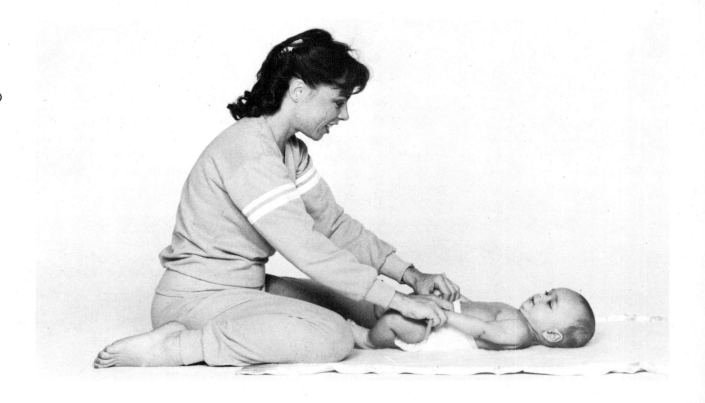

keeps his shoulder muscles flexible, too.

2.

Slowly raise your baby's hands over his head. Then bring them back to their original position. Repeat the sequence 16 times.

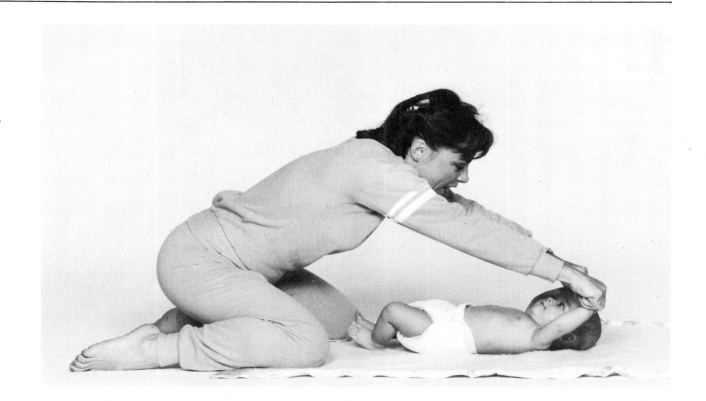

Sit-Up with Dowel

This exercise is excellent for hand, arm, and shoulder strength and for the abdominal muscles. If you don't have a dowel, simply hold your baby's hands.

1.

Place your baby on his back and have him grasp a dowel in both hands. Cover his hands with your fingers to secure his grip.

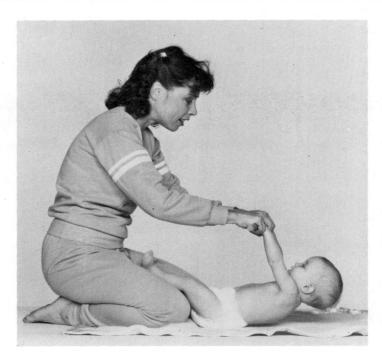

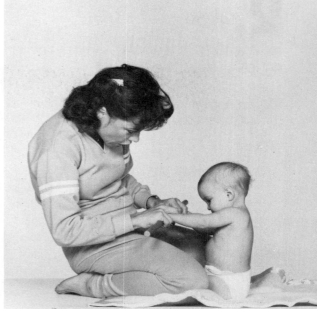

2.

Slowly pull the dowel
toward you so that your
baby comes up into a
sitting position. Allow
your baby to sit, and
reposition his hands if
necessary.

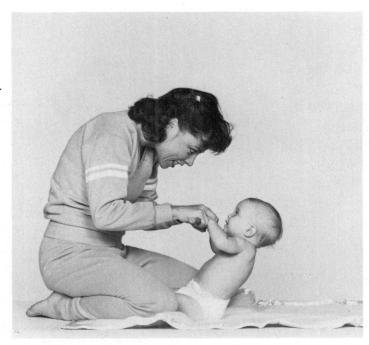

3.

Then slowly lower your
baby to the original
position. Repeat the
sequence 4 times.

Pillow Crawl

Not only does this exercise enhance strength and coordination, it fosters curiosity and the ability to accept and master challenges.

1.

Place a pillow on the floor and your baby on his tummy on top of it. Your baby's hands should be resting on the floor in front of the pillow.

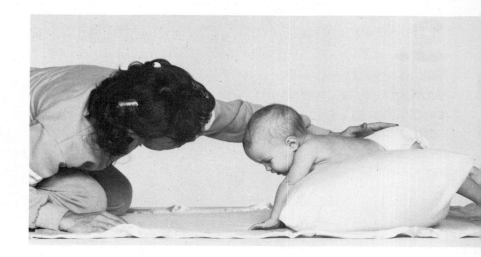

2.

Coax your baby forward, boosting him a bit as he inches over the pillow. Keep your other hand near your baby's shoulders.

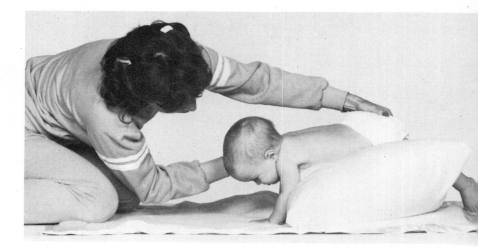

3.

Talk to your baby as he works his way over the pillow. Repeat the sequence 4 times.

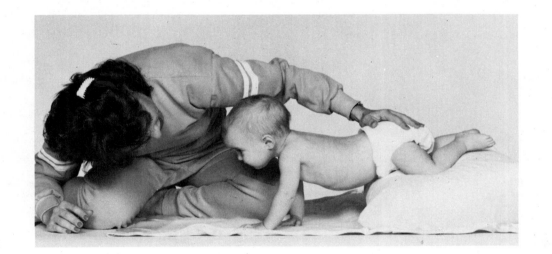

Toddlers:
12 to 22 Months

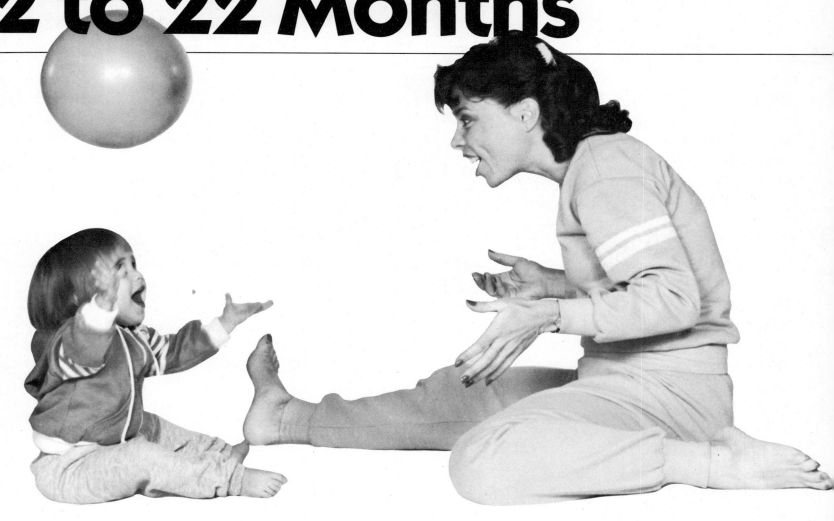

Where did all his energy come from? From now on, when your child is awake, he will be on the go. And go he does–crawling, walking, running in almost every direction at once. From room to room, obstacle to obstacle, no to no. Walking into furniture and knocking over lamps seem to be the norm at this stage. Bumps, bruises, and spills are the order of the day.

How do you cope? With patience, determination–and exercise. Exercise can help channel some of your baby's energy. What's more, through exercise you can teach your child to use his body correctly so he has more control while he is racing from one new experience to the next.

Your child is constantly learning. Some days, 40 minutes of exercise isn't long enough; on other days, 15 minutes is too long. And there are days when your child just won't feel like doing a thing. Don't force him into experiences he doesn't want or isn't ready for. He needs time to digest all the things he's already learned. We use vacations for this. Toddlers use a few hours or a day here and there. During these periods, children are processing what they have learned so that they will have room inside to learn the next thing.

Sleep, too, is critical to children of this age. They often don't stop until they have used up all their energy and have nothing left to go on. Toddlers who must function past the point of tiredness become cranky and impossible—and rightfully so. Very often, a short catnap will totally refresh and invigorate a child. So give your child the rest he needs when he needs it.

Nothing seems safe with the advent of walking, be it at 10, 14, or even 18 months of age. Your baby is now a very curious little person with, it seems to you, no sense of reasoning. But it's really not a question of "no reasoning" here. His perception is simply different from yours. His mental vocabulary hasn't put a judgment, a value, on anything yet. As far as a toddler of this age is concerned, if he can see it, he can have it. If he can reach it, it's to be touched. If he can get it into his mouth, it's to be tasted. The chair you sit on is the chair to be climbed on. The outlet you plug the lamp into is to be explored. The door that is opened is to be closed. Your child is experimenting with the world around him in every way he physically and mentally can. He must get to know his new world; he's going to be living in it the rest of his life.

What does this have to do with exercise? By exercising your toddler every day, you are teaching him how to control his body. He will become not only stronger but more coordinated as well—which means he'll have fewer spills and scrapes.

The most important and neglected part of the body is the abdominal muscles. These, along with the lower back muscles, control the body. If the abdominals aren't functioning properly, the rest of the body will not function as well as it could. Therefore, Roll-Downs should be done daily. It will be difficult at first, unless your child has been doing it all along. But in time, he will become quite proficient at it. Watch how his other movements change and become smoother as he develops strong abdominals.

There is so much to see and to do that your baby doesn't hold on to a thought for more than 15 or 30 seconds before something new sparks his interest. This is as it should be. Take this into account when you exercise your child, and switch exercises every 10 or 15 seconds. This not only increases coordination, but it avoids injury, too. While one area of the body is working, another is resting. Therefore, muscles don't get sore. Alternating the exercises is also important for developing coordination, teaching the body and mind to respond quickly and effectively. Alternating between the

Monkey Walk and the Frog Hop exercises will seem impossible in the beginning, but notice how well-coordinated your child becomes when you keep at it! By doing the strengthening as well as the coordination-enhancing exercises, you will notice a difference in your child's behavior as he races from situation to situation.

Your child will sometimes follow directions at this age. But don't become flustered if nine times out of ten he won't. There's so much going on in his mind that he may not be able to respond to your request. Instead of asking or telling your child to do an exercise and getting frustrated when he won't, do it with him. This can be fun for both of you, and keeps the stress level down.

At times, it may seem as if your child is making no progress. His muscles just don't seem to want to work. And his brain doesn't seem to be functioning at all. Nothing seems connected. Don't be discouraged. This is known as a plateau, and your child is, in a sense, resting. Just as your child goes through growth spurts and then non-growth periods, he goes through learning spurts and resting periods. He's catching up with himself and preparing for the next step forward. Keep offering the information: when your child is ready, he will take it.

I have included various types of equipment in this program that I have found to be helpful, safe, and fun. A ladder, for example, is a versatile piece of equipment. And it is especially fun if there is something waiting for them at the other end: a tambourine, say, or a favorite toy. As the child begins to walk, walking between the rungs enhances leg strength and, of course, coordination. Soon the child can move from one end to the other, stepping on each rung. Eventually, one end of the ladder can be raised and the child can climb from low end to high end.

The challenge of mastering equipment can teach patience, too. Some children will spend an entire half hour on one piece of equipment until they master it. In subsequent sessions, they can go back to this first difficult and successful experience to remind themselves of how good it felt to accomplish the task and to rejoice in how easy it is to do now.

The equipment I suggest in this book is just the beginning. If you can think of new and exciting things to add, do so! It is important now to add as much equipment as possible to your exercise program. I have included the ladder, a raised two-by-four, and a balloon. Use these if you can or make up exercises with other things you may have inside or outside your home.

The clothes your toddler exercises in are not important. He (or you) may like the idea of a sweat suit. But when your infant is crawling on the ramp or another piece of equipment, I suggest that he crawl on bare knees and exercise on bare feet. After all, his toes have to get a workout, too.

Again, as you did when he was an infant, work to or with music when you exercise your toddler. And if a record or the radio is playing when he is alone, notice his response. Music speaks to children. They will move naturally according to the tempo of the music. Exercising to music augments this natural rhythm, and their movements will soon be rhythmic even when they are not listening to music. Fast or slow, their actions will be smooth. This inner rhythm and coordination will last for life.

Forty-five minutes is a good period of time for your child's exercise program. Again, this may be too long on some days, or if your child is going through a real spurt, too short. You will know by the way your child responds. The time of day is unimportant. Choose an hour that is comfortable for both of you.

Arm Crossovers

Holding your toddler close to you is a cozy, encouraging position from which to do exercises. This exercise is not only excellent for your toddler's flexibility

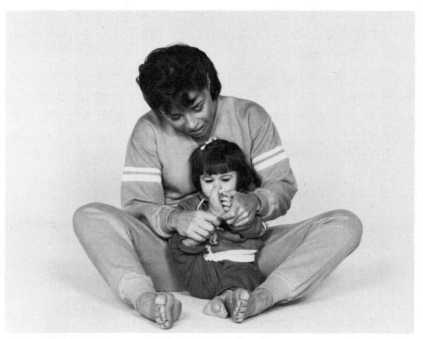

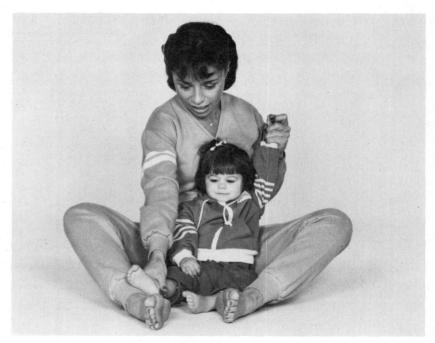

1. Have your toddler sit on the floor between your legs so that he can lean back on your stomach. Grasp his right ankle and left hand and bring the foot and hand together.

2. Stretch your toddler's right leg out and his left arm high over his head. Repeat this sequence 4 times with each opposite hand and foot.

and coordination but it also strengthens arms, legs, shoulders, and upper back.

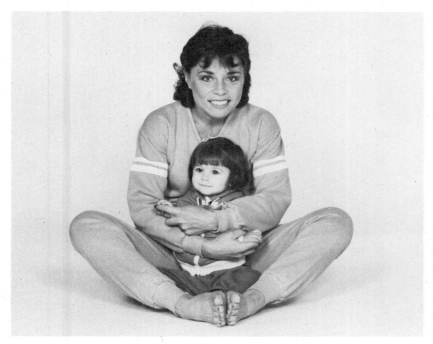

3. Now hold your toddler's wrists and hands in yours, and cross his arms across his chest.

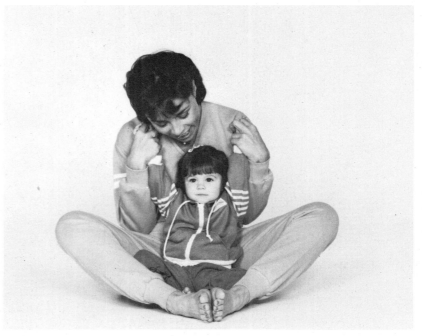

4. Slowly stretch both of your toddler's arms above his head. Then return them to cross in front of his chest again. Repeat this sequence 4 times.

Arm Swings

This exercise is excellent for loosening tight shoulder and torso muscles as well as for strengthening abdominal and waist muscles. Try to keep your arms at

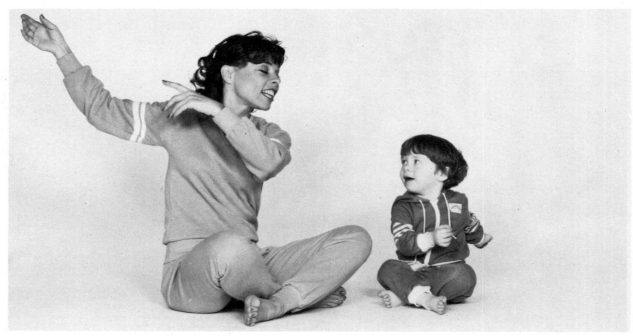

1. Sit on the floor next to each other with your legs crossed in front of you. Swing both of your arms to one side, at shoulder height.

shoulder height and your buttocks on the
floor. Circulation will be enhanced while
tension is released in the upper back,
shoulders, and neck.

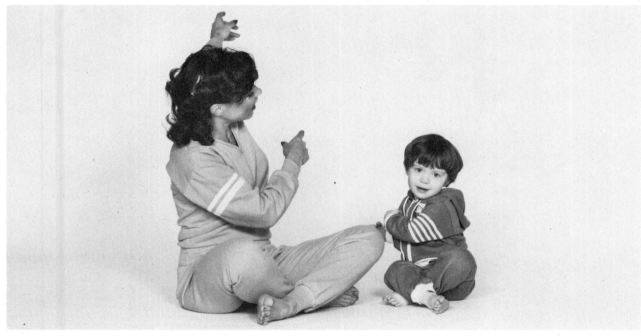

2. Swing your arms to the
other side. Repeat the
sequence 16 times,
keeping a fluid motion.

Forehead-to-Toes

Your toddler will enjoy trying to touch his head to his toes. The more he does this exercise, the closer he will be able to bring his forehead to his toes. This

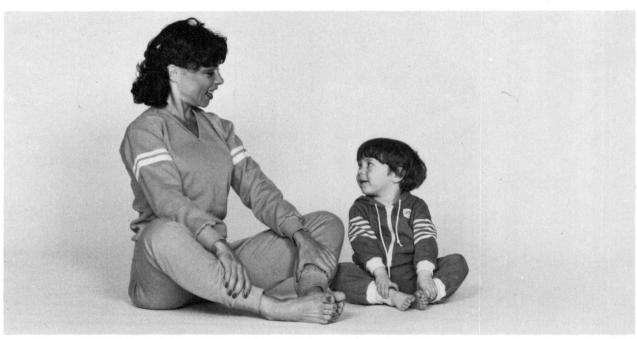

1. Sit next to each other on the floor with your feet together, knees bent and apart, and ankles or calves clasped in your hands.

exercise is particularly good for lower back flexibility as well as for abdominal strength.

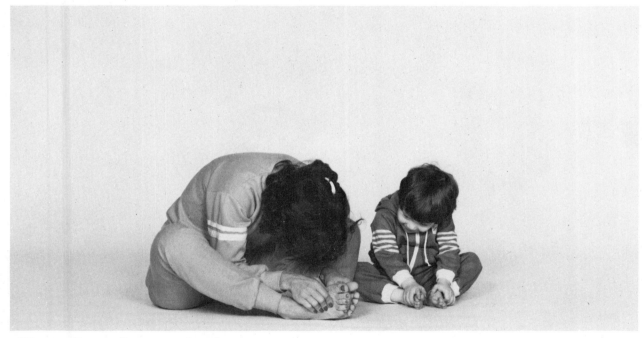

2. Rounding your back, gently pull your head down toward your toes. Return to the original position. Repeat the sequence 16 times.

Roll-Downs

Doing a proper sit-up is still a long time away; in the meantime, Roll-Downs are a great way of increasing abdominal strength in your youngster. Make sure

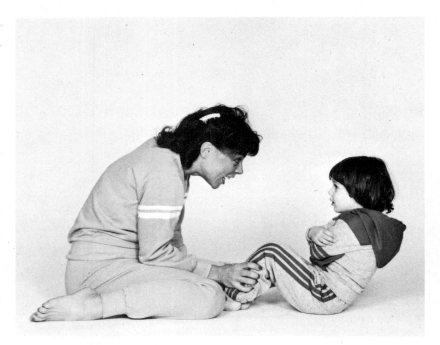

1. Sit facing your toddler. Have your toddler sit with his knees bent, feet flat on the floor, and his arms crossed on his chest.

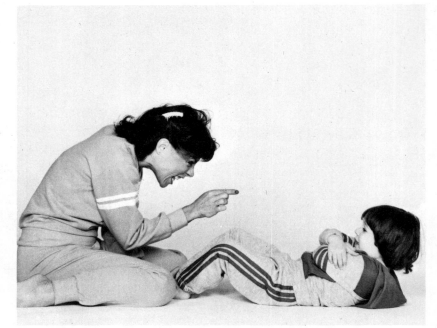

2. Holding your toddler's ankles so that his knees remain bent and his feet stay on the floor, have him slowly lie down on his back to the count of 4.

your toddler rounds his back as he lowers it to the floor. He should also try to lower his body without leaning to one side or the other.

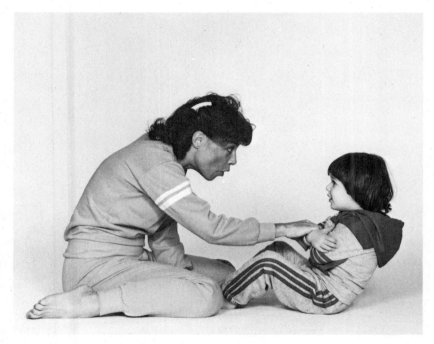

3. Have your toddler return to the sitting position, using his hands or having you pull him up. Repeat the sequence 4 to 8 times.

Raising the Flag

Not only are the pectorals and inner arms made more flexible with this exercise, they are strengthened as well. Keep both arms as straight as possible.

1.

Get down on your hands and knees next to each other, with your backs parallel to the floor.

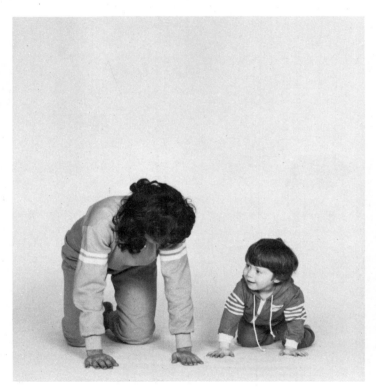
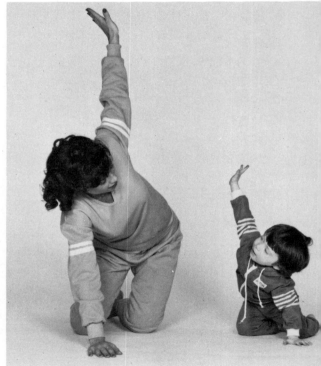

2.

Keeping one hand on the floor and your arm straight, raise the other arm as high as possible.

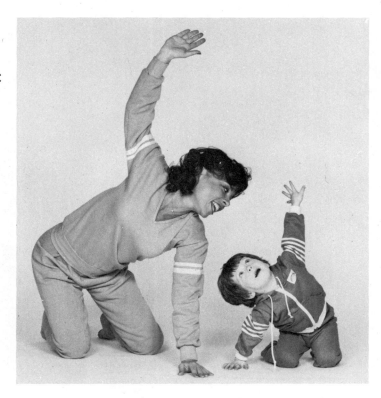

3.

Lower your raised hand to the floor, keeping your arm straight, then raise your other arm, elbow straight, as high as possible. Then lower it. Repeat the sequence 8 times.

The Squat

The entire leg, especially thighs and knees, gets a good workout during this exercise. Lower your bottom as close to the floor as possible when you squat.

1.

Stand next to each other with your feet slightly apart and your hands on your hips.

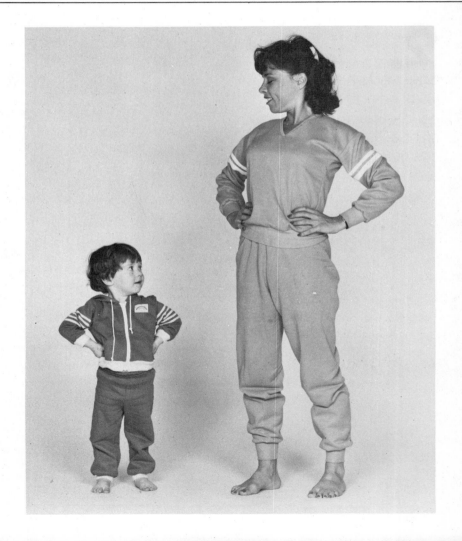

2.

Squat down as low as you can and place your hands on the floor in front of you. Stand up again and repeat the sequence 8 times.

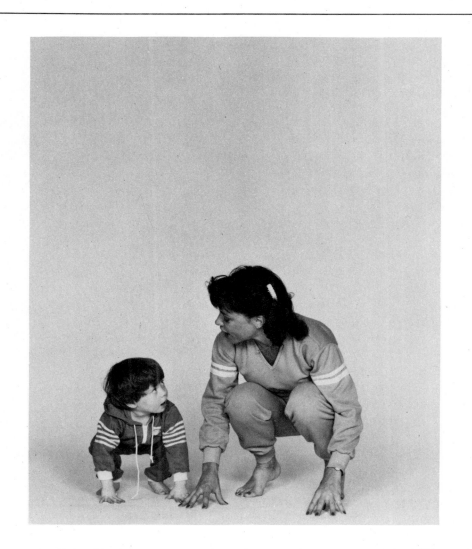

Monkey Walk

Children love to move around, and incorporating play movements into exercises makes them even more fun. Having your child go through your legs

1.

Get on your hands and feet, keeping your legs as straight as possible. Lean your weight forward so that it is evenly distributed between your hands and feet. Have your toddler take the same position.

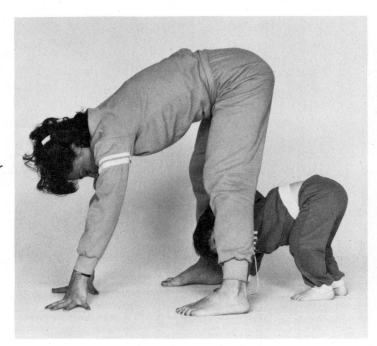
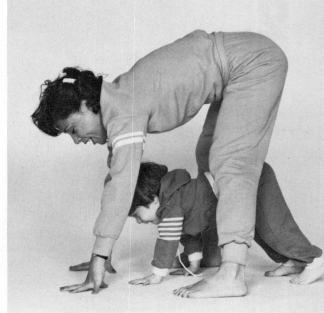

enhances concentration. This exercise is excellent for shoulder, arm, and upper back strength as well as lower back and hamstring flexibility.

2.

Have your toddler "monkey walk" through your legs and arms on his hands and feet. . .

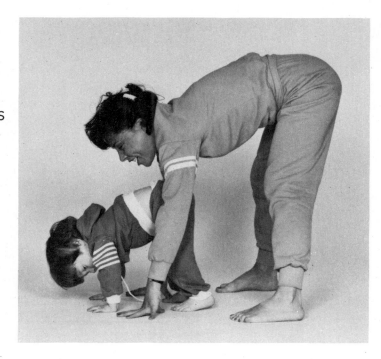

3.

. . . until he comes out in front of you. Repeat the sequence at least twice.

Rabbit Hop

This exercise is excellent for coordination and strengthening legs. Be careful not to bump into each other as you hop around the room!

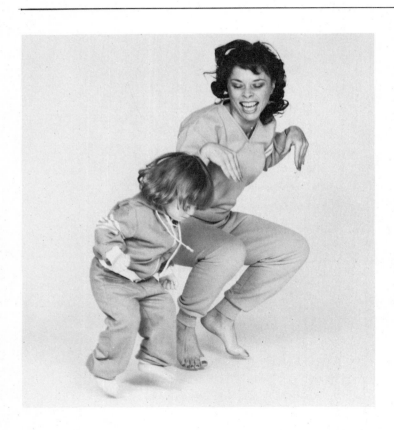

Squat down with your toddler and pull your hands up in front of your chest. Hop around the room in this posture, squatting as low as you can when you land each time.

Duck Walk

This exercise strengthens leg muscles and encourages coordination. Vocal cords will get a workout too, if you quack while you waddle.

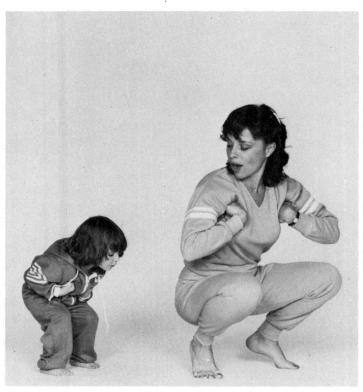

1. Squat down with your toddler and bend your elbows, placing your hands under your arms.

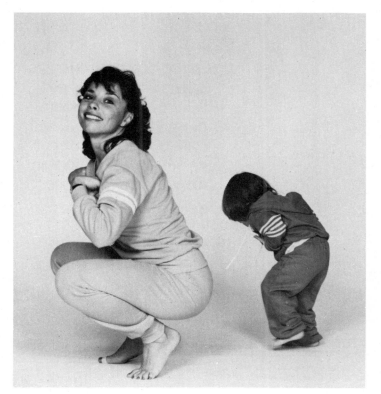

2. Keeping your knees bent and your bottom close to the floor, waddle around the room, moving one foot at a time.

Frog Hop

It may take a little while for your toddler to coordinate his hands and feet for this exercise, but mastery will come with repetition and patience. The Frog Hop is

1.

Squat down next to each other, with your knees bent and your bottom close to the floor. Reach out and place your hands approximately a foot in front of you (6 inches for your toddler).

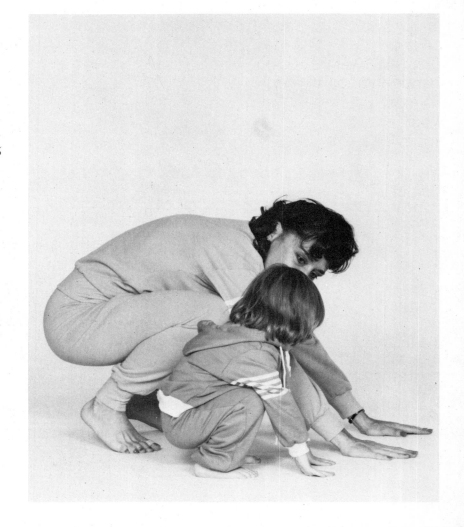

excellent for arms, shoulders, and legs.

2.

Lean your weight on your hands and hop forward to meet your hands with your feet. Hop across the room in this manner.

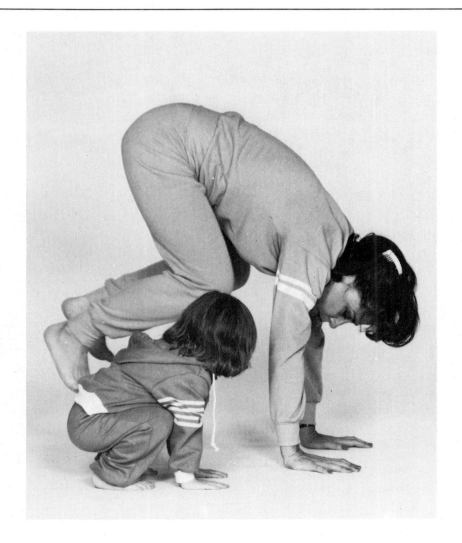

Catch-a-Balloon

Children love this exercise. It allows them to improve their concentration and eye-hand coordination while having a wonderful time.

1.

Sit facing your toddler and hold a big, brightly colored balloon in front of you. Roll the balloon toward your child. Have your toddler roll or throw the balloon back to you. If the balloon goes flying across the room, have your toddler fetch it. It is fun for him and saves you wear and tear. Repeat the sequence 8 times.

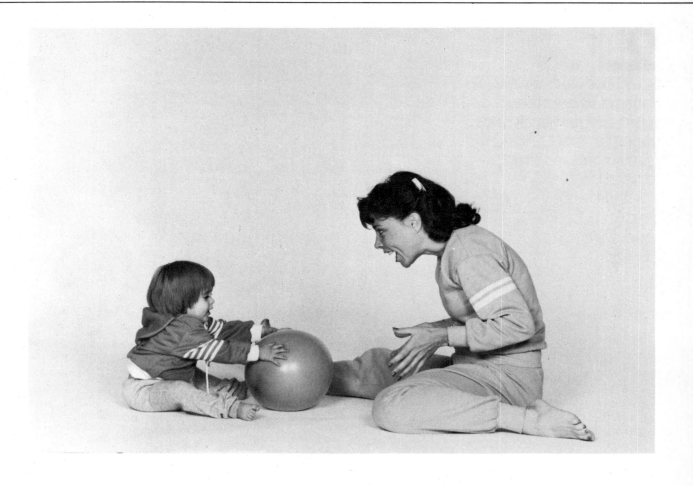

2.

Now have your child sit a few feet away from you while you stand and hold the balloon out to him. Throw the balloon gently to your child. Have your child throw or roll the balloon back to you, and repeat the sequence 8 times.

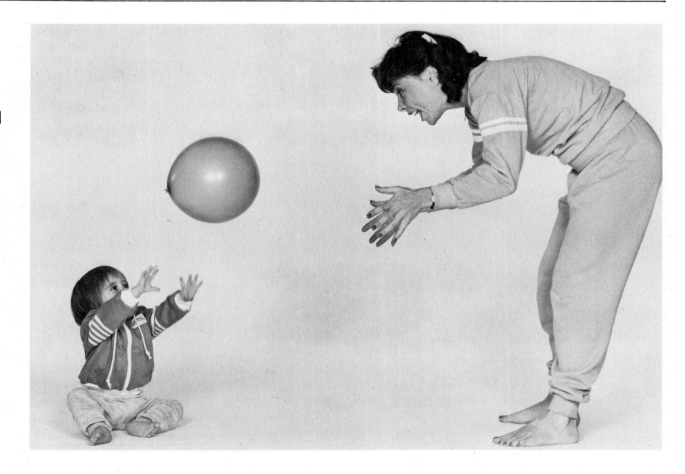

Walking the Plank

Balance is very important for comfortable movement in general. Walking on the "low, straight, and narrow" enhances eye-foot coordination,

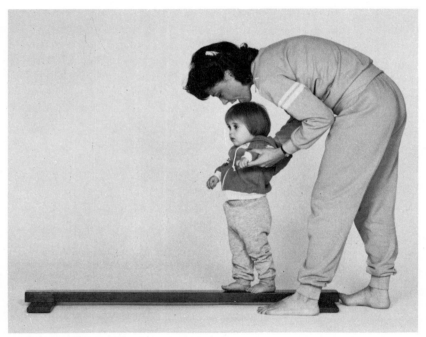

1. Place a raised two-by-four on the floor and put your child at one end with both feet on the board, one in front of the other.

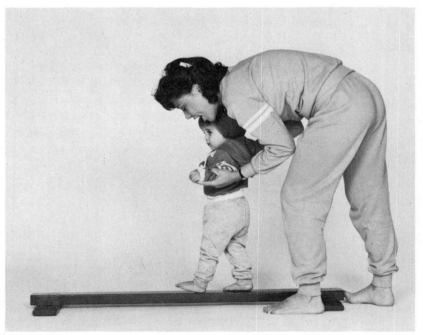

2. Stand at your child's side and hold his left hand while placing your right hand under his arm.

and helps develop a sense of balance.

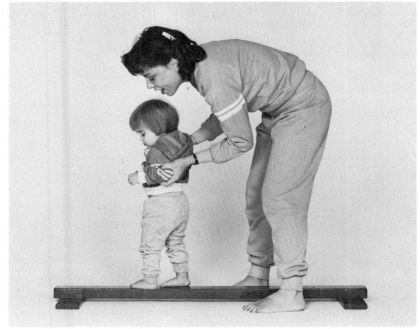

3. Have your toddler walk from one end of the board to the other, telling him which foot he is stepping forward on as he goes. Repeat the sequence 4 times, twice in each direction.

Plank Wheelbarrow

When first doing this exercise, be sure you support your toddler's lower back by holding him under both his legs and chest. As he gains in strength and

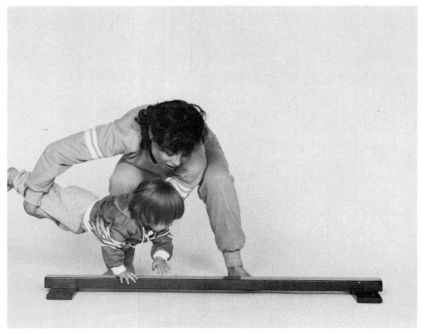

1. Place a raised two-by-four on the floor, and have your toddler place his hands on the board while you hold his legs and chest.

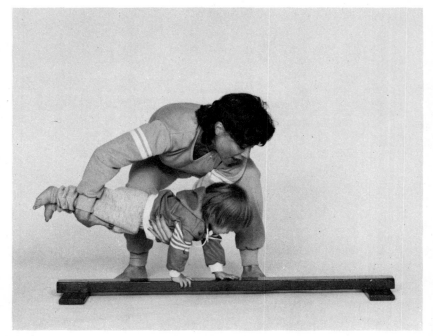

2. Slowly coax your child forward, having him place one hand in front of the other. Tell him which hand he is using as he goes.

confidence, you can move your hands to support only his hips and then even further to hold him by the upper thighs. Eye-hand coordination is the main benefit of this exercise, but it also helps strengthen the arms, shoulders, chest, and back muscles.

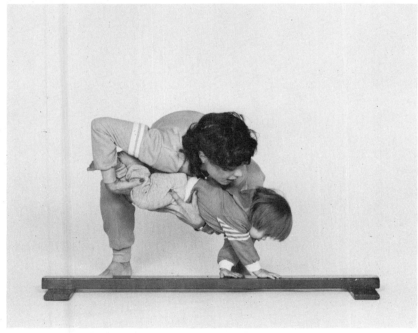

3. "Walk" your toddler from one end of the board to the other. Repeat the sequence 4 times, twice in each direction.

Train Track Traverse

This exercise enhances your child's coordination, for he must look and be careful of where he is putting his feet and hands. Leg, abdominal, and lower back

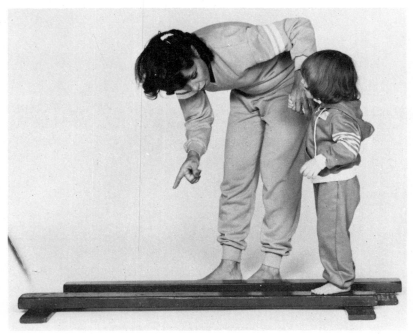

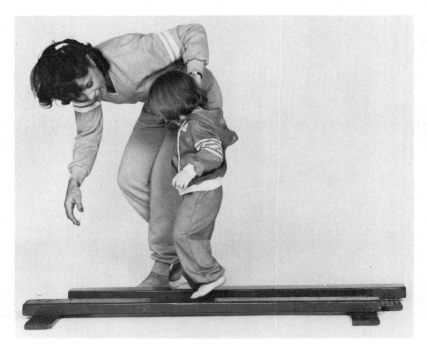

1. Place 2 two-by-fours on the floor, approximately 1 foot apart and parallel to each other. Have your toddler stand at one end with one foot placed on each board.

2. Hold your toddler's hand and have him walk forward, placing his left foot on the left board and his right foot on the right board, traversing the length of the boards. Repeat the sequence 4 times.

muscles are strengthened in the process.
The 2-by-4's used in this (and any
other) exercise may be raised, or placed
flat on the floor.

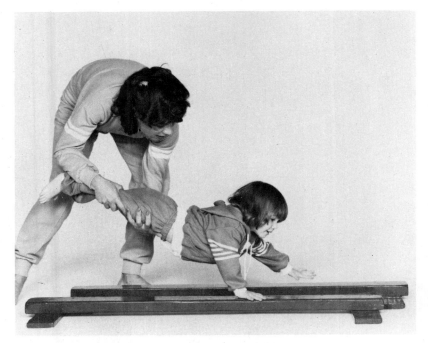

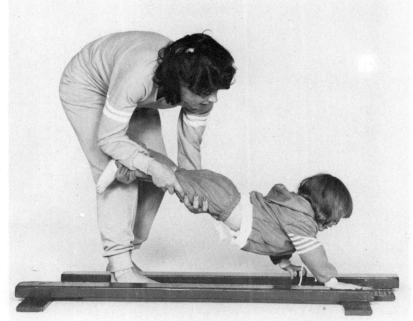

3. Then have your toddler place one of his hands near the end of each board. Hold your toddler's thighs and legs so that his feet are off the floor and his weight is resting on his hands.

4. Have your child "walk" the length of the boards on his hands, placing his right hand on the right board and his left hand on the left board as he goes. Repeat the sequence 4 times.

Ladder Climb

Eye-hand coordination and total motor development are enhanced in this exercise. Your toddler will have an easy time coordinating his arms, but his legs

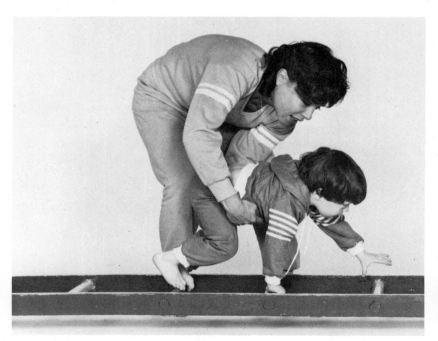

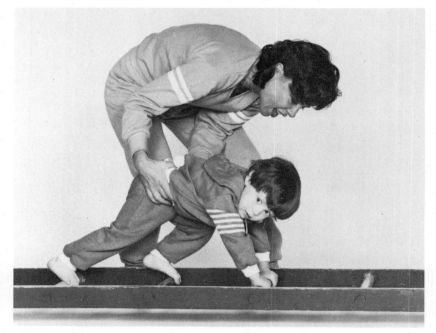

1. Place a ladder on the floor and have your child put his feet on the last rung and his hands in front of him on the next rung. Grasp him around his hips.

2. Have your toddler reach for each rung, first with one hand and then the other, with his feet following for the entire length of the ladder. Repeat this sequence 4 times.

will take a little more time and practice. Tell him which hand he is using as he goes, and be sure he alternates. For the second half of this exercise, raise and securely prop one end of the ladder 3 feet off the floor.

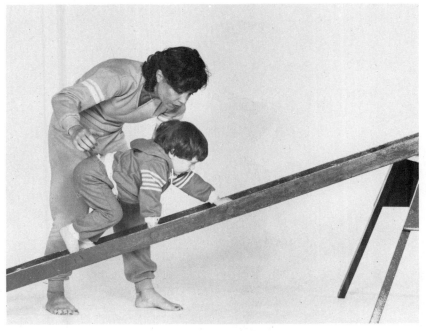

3. With the ladder raised, have your toddler place his feet on the lowest rung and his hands on the next rung. Keep one hand close to his hips and the other near his chest.

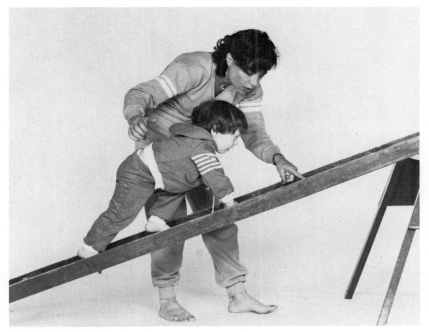

4. Have your toddler reach for each rung, first with his left hand and then his right. Coax him up the ladder, with his right and left feet following his hands. Repeat the sequence 4 times.

Toddlers: 23 Months to 3 Years

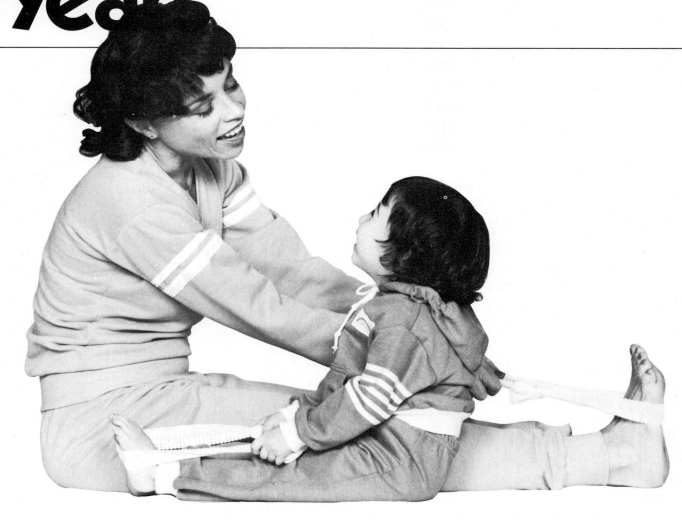

And you thought you knew your toddler. What a surprise package he is! He is definitely his own person now—with likes and dislikes, good moods and bad, yeses and nos.

Up to now, your child believed he was the only center of the universe, with the world at his beck and call. Now he's discovering he's not the center of things. The world no longer comes to the toddler; the toddler must go to the world.

This may seem obvious to you. After all, you've known it for years. But your toddler hasn't. Remember: all of his needs have been met, every desire fulfilled. Why should this now be an issue? After all, the things that seem so important to reach were there before. But your child's attention span is now longer and his physical capabilities are greater. He holds on to thoughts and loves to solve problems. If climbing onto a counter seems like a good idea, he will find a way to do it. No matter where you put him, he will hold that counter in his mind for quite some time, and he will continue to try to figure out a way to get to the top of it. It's a place to explore, and his well-coordinated little body is going to get him up there.

Now is the time when you may wonder why you helped him become so well-coordinated in the first place! If he weren't so agile, you might think, he might not attempt that counter climb. But this is not so. He'd try because it's there, no matter what physical shape he's in. The difference between an exercised baby and one who's not is that the exercised, coordinated child will climb with greater ease—and more safety.

Your child is now physically strong and has a good memory. Therefore, you have not only a curious bolt of lightning on your hands, but very often a mule as well. This is a wonderful sign. It means that your child has grown in intelligence and physical dexterity. All you have to do is survive when he's either exploring or turning his mind and body toward getting something you don't want him to have.

He also has a strong will. He wants things his way. This is a mixed blessing. The good news is that he will use his imagination in all sorts of new ways to get what he wants. Not only will he use his body, but he will actually create physical apparatus and use it to achieve his goal. The bad news is he'll get there. So be on guard!

Now is the time for you to use as much equipment

as you can in your program. If you started using equipment before your child could walk, that equipment is still fine. But you must use your imagination to keep it interesting for your child. Whereas before the boards were low to the ground, now they should be three feet off the ground. At first your child may be frightened. Don't force him to climb onto the raised boards or balance beam. Hold him there a few seconds and then put him back on the floor. As his fear dissipates, you can help him walk from one end to the other.

Start using some new equipment, too. Why not try Frisbees, for example? They are a wonderful way to enhance concentration, eye and hand coordination, and muscle strength. Try doing Squatting Knee Bends with Frisbees, reaching high and then touching them to the floor. You will be amazed at how your child's coordination and concentration develop just through using this simple piece of equipment. They are also fun to work with.

Equipment can also help teach a child right from left. If he uses the left foot when you've asked for the right and you tell him "wrong foot," your child will change to the right one. If you don't bother to explain this to him, he won't know the difference. I recommend that you start teaching him the difference between right and left as soon as possible.

I have included the use of a dowel, a sawhorse (raised beam), a ramp, and straps in this section. Use other apparatus from previous sections or ideas you come up with at home as well. Be inventive. Your child will benefit.

In this or anything else, be consistent. But know that your child won't be—not now, anyway. He may know right and left, but that doesn't mean he'll use the knowledge. He likes to have things his own way, and he's testing himself and you to see how far he can go. This is where difficulties arise. Just as there are days when everything pleases him, there are days when nothing makes him happy, when he's totally contrary. Exercising should be fun. If it becomes a battle of two wills, both are going to lose. Rather than fight to get through an exercise, change it. Come back to the first one later on, or even on a different day.

Toddlers love a reaction. They need positive reinforcement. So praise him frequently. The more you show him how wonderfully he is doing, the better he'll do. Toddlers also love to succeed. They love to set goals and then accomplish what they set out to do. Watch a child take apart a toy and try to put it back together again!

Learning new tricks is exciting; repeating old ones is reassuring. Children are always ready to learn something new. Just remember that they love repetition, too. It makes them feel secure, and become more sure in their movements. There is nothing worse than wanting to do a new trick and not having the foundation on which to take that next step. It may seem boring to you, but your child must learn all the basics first, until those basic moves are second nature. After they become second nature, the sky is the limit, and his body is safely prepared to take him where he wants to go.

As I mentioned before, children sometimes develop different fears at this age. Don't force your child to do something he is afraid of. Fears pass. If, for example, your child develops a fear of heights, hold him closely, for a short period of time, while he stands on something high. Reassure him and help him to feel safe. After all, even though *you* know he's fine, his fear is very real. Forcing him to do something he is afraid of is counterproductive.

As his fear lessens, you can gradually let go of him, and lengthen his stay up there until you are holding him by the hand and he can move comfortably along. This technique should be used whenever your child is frightened. His fears will dissipate quickly, and he will feel wonderful as he masters each. As he learns he is in control, he will begin to master those little terrors on his own, and his self-confidence will grow. As this grows, so will his self-esteem.

Choose a time when your child is usually active to exercise. If you wait until he's too tired, the exercise session, which can and should be loving, will turn out badly. There's always tomorrow—just don't let too many todays pass. Exercise with your child several times a week for various periods of time. Try to get at least one 45-minute period in per week. The rest of the sessions can vary according to mood and schedule.

Clothing is not important here, although be aware that children love special clothes for special activities. Let your child start to decide what music he'd like to use. Guide him, of course, but also give him the opportunity to choose his own favorites.

Squatting Knee Bend

This classic exercise is one your child should do daily. It strengthens the entire leg and is especially good for the knees.

1.

Stand next to each other with your feet slightly apart and your hands on your hips.

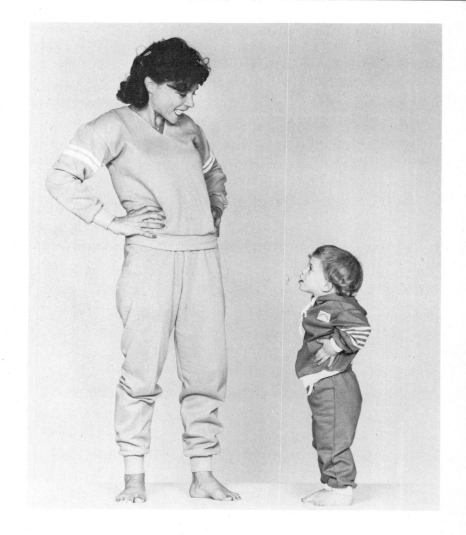

2.◆

Bend your knees to a squat position with your bottom close to the floor. Hold for 4 seconds before you stand up again. Repeat the sequence 8 times.

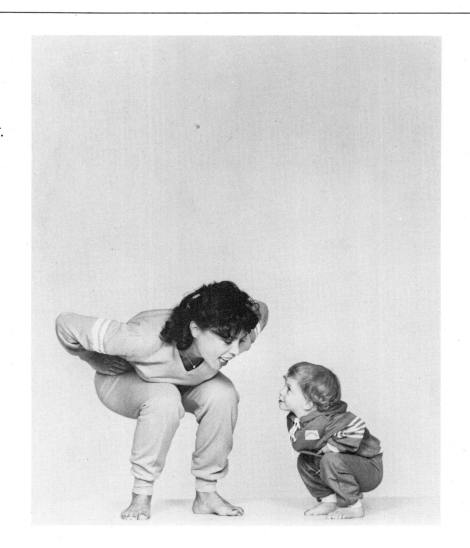

The Pretzel

This seemingly silly exercise firms up abdominal muscles, while at the same time enhancing leg and lower back flexibility.

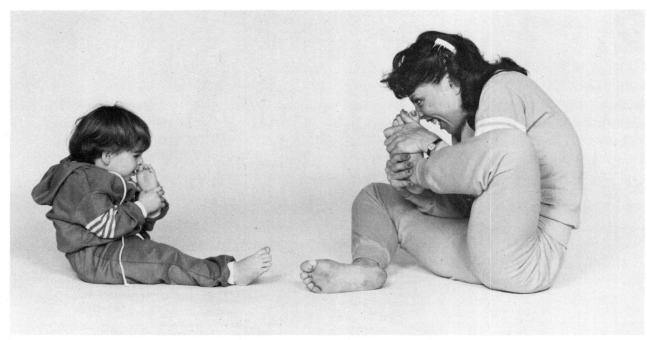

1. Sit near each other with your legs stretched out on the floor in front of you. Hold your left foot with both hands and raise it up to touch your nose. Lower it to the ground.

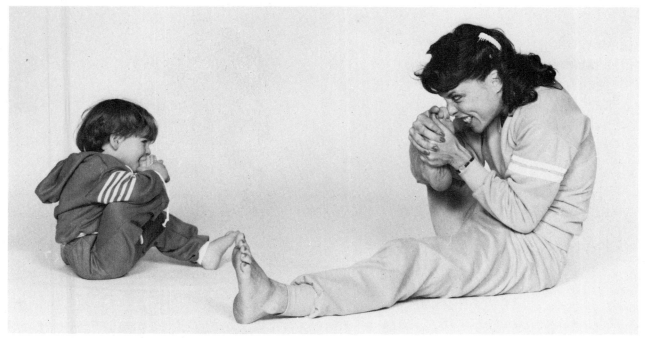

2. Now hold your right foot with both hands and raise it up to your nose. Repeat the sequence 12 times.

The Jack Rabbit

This exercise is great fun, and gives the quadriceps (thigh muscles) a tremendous workout. To get the most benefit from it, squat as low as you can

1.

Stand next to each other with feet slightly apart. Squat down, placing your hands on the floor in front of you.

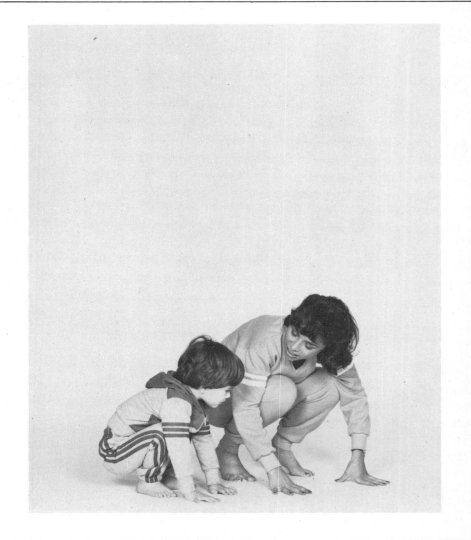

and jump as high as possible.

2.

Spring up as high as you can, straightening your body as much as possible while you are in the air. Land in the squat position. Repeat the sequence 4 to 8 times.

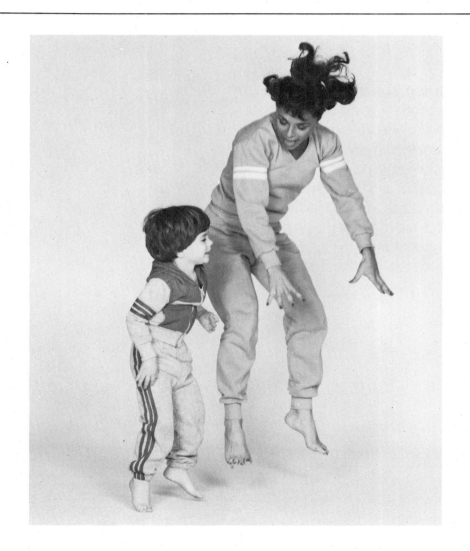

Arm Swings with Dowel

When you and your toddler hold a dowel between you, you and he will be pulling against each other. This steady resistance is excellent for

1.

Sit with your legs crossed, facing your child. Hold a dowel between you, placing your hands over your toddler's. Swing the dowel as far to your left and his right as possible without lifting your buttocks off the floor.

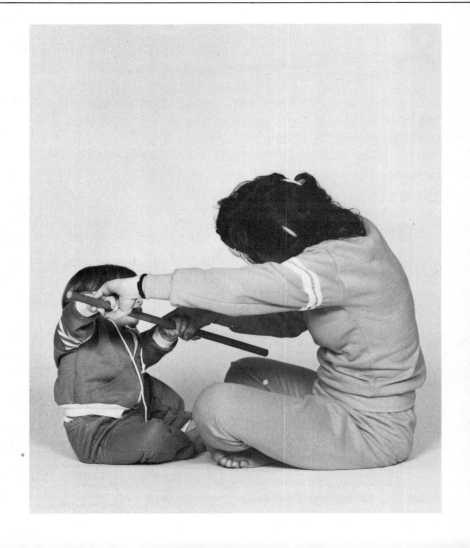

developing coordination as well as for strengthening the arms, midriff, chest, back, and abdominal muscles.

2.

Then swing the dowel to your right and his left. Repeat the sequence 16 times, keeping your movements fluid and regular.

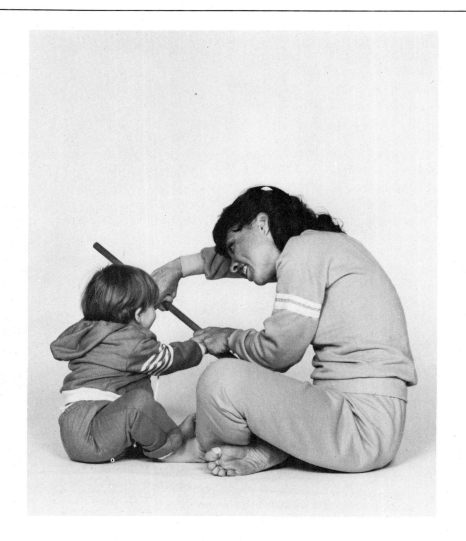

Sit Up and Stand

Using a dowel for this exercise builds strength in your child's arms as well as his abdominal muscles.

1.

Have your toddler lie on his back and hold a dowel with both hands. Place your hands over his to ensure his grip. Kneel at his calves, with your legs on either side of his legs, and grip them with your knees.

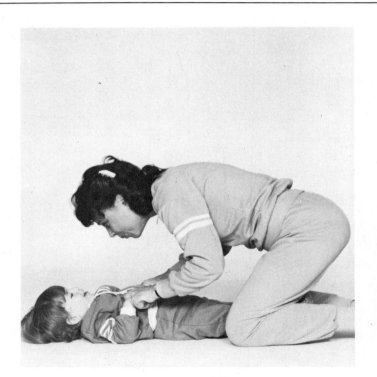

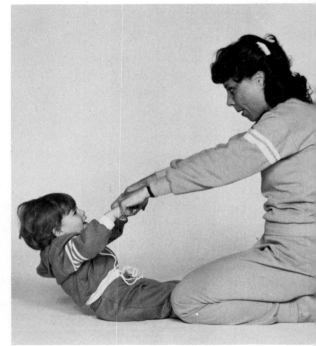

2.

Slowly pull your toddler up into a sitting position.

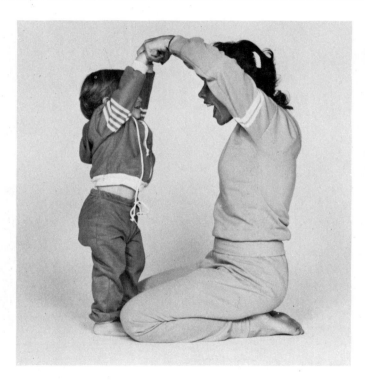

3.

Raise your toddler's arms above his head and pull him up to a standing position. Repeat the sequence 4 times.

Row Your Boat

This exercise is excellent for arm, back, chest, and abdominal strength as well as hamstring flexibility. Keep your legs as straight as possible.

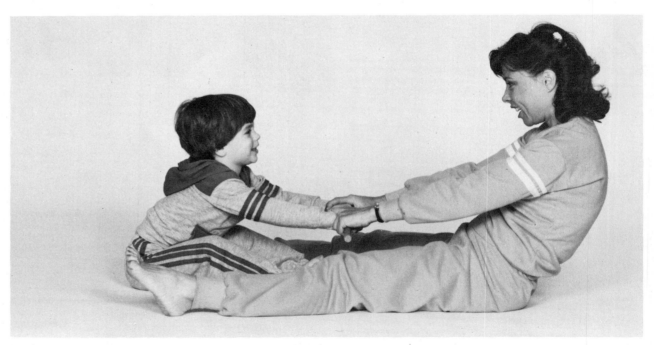

1. Sit facing your child with your legs apart and your child's feet braced on the insides of your knees. Clasp a dowel between you with your hands over his. Lean backward, pulling your toddler forward.

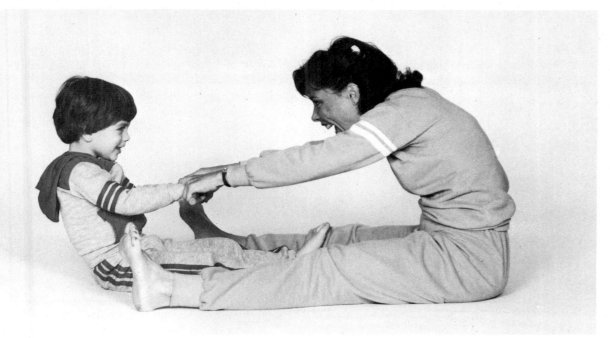

2. Then have your toddler lean backward, pulling you forward. Be sure to keep your legs straight. Repeat the sequence 16 times.

Dowel Hang

This exercise not only increases hand strength, it also increases strength in the arms, shoulders, chest, and upper back as well as in the abdominals and

1.

Stand facing your toddler and have him grasp a dowel in both hands. Cover his hands with yours to ensure his grip.

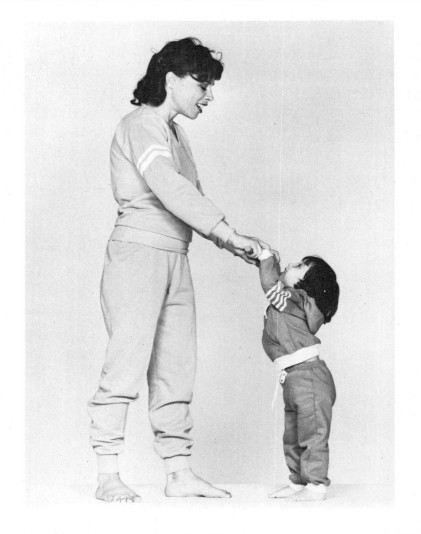

the lower back. After your toddler is comfortable with this exercise, have him bring his knees up to his chest a few times during each hang (not shown here).

2.

Keeping your hands over your toddler's, slowly lift him into the air and then lower him again. Repeat the sequence 4 times.

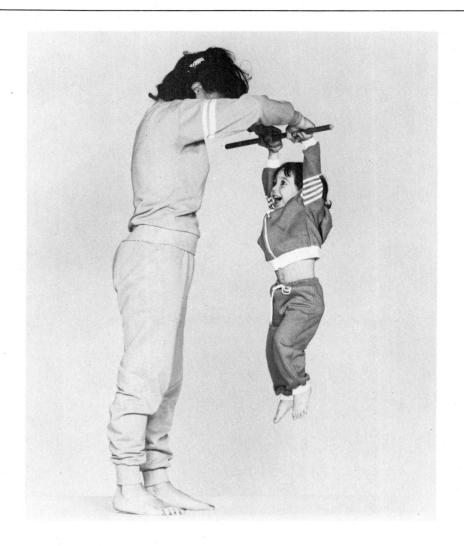

Flexibility Pull

Pulling your torso forward with a strap looped around the soles of your feet increases hamstring flexibility. You and your toddler must be fully warmed up

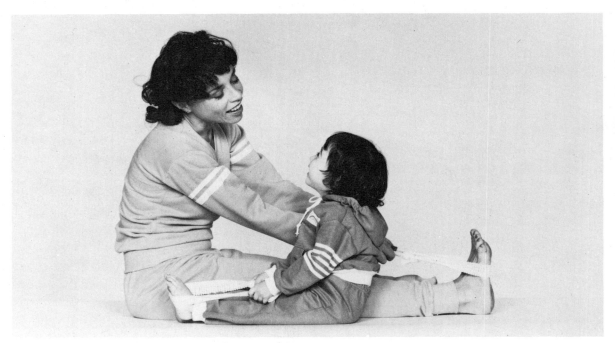

1. Sit on the floor facing each other with your legs stretched straight out in front of you. Hold a towel or strap in both hands and loop it over both feet, which remain together.

before doing this exercise, since you will
be really stretching your hamstrings.

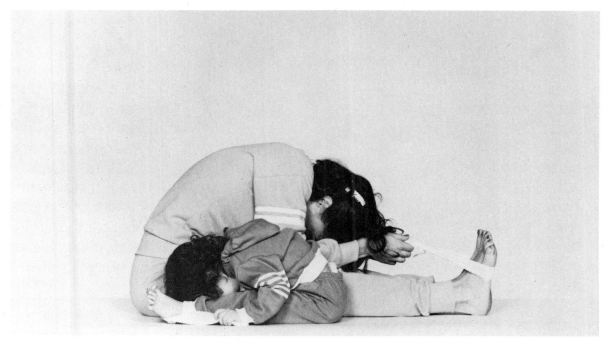

2. Keeping your legs straight
and feet together, pull
your head down to your
knees and then sit up
straight again. Repeat the
sequence 8 to 16 times.

Balance Beam Walk

If you've been following the program in this book, your toddler has experience walking on a 2-by-4 close to the floor. Now it's time to introduce him to a higher

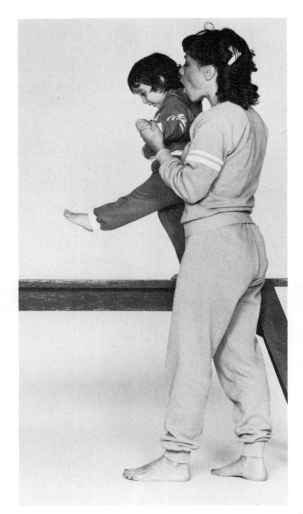

1.

Place your toddler at one end of a 4-inch-wide saw-horse or balance beam. Standing on your toddler's left, clasp his left hand in yours. Put your right arm around his back and grasp his right arm. Have your toddler take a step forward, using his left foot first. Tell him which foot it is.

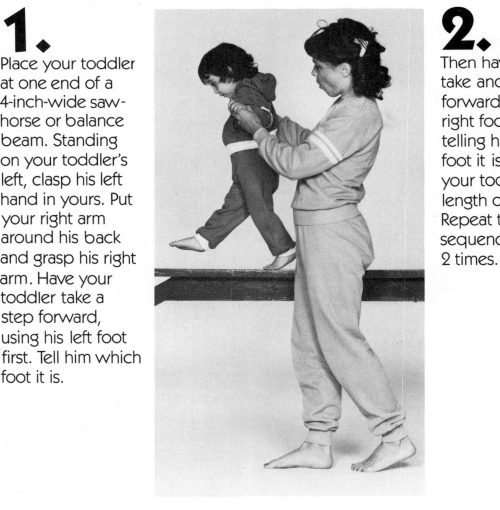

2.

Then have him take another step forward with his right foot, again telling him which foot it is. "Walk" your toddler the length of the beam. Repeat this sequence at least 2 times.

structure. He may experience some fear in the beginning, so stay close until he feels secure. As he feels more comfortable, he will need you less and less. Just be sure to be there if he does. This exercise is excellent for balance, poise, and coordination, and enhances self-confidence.

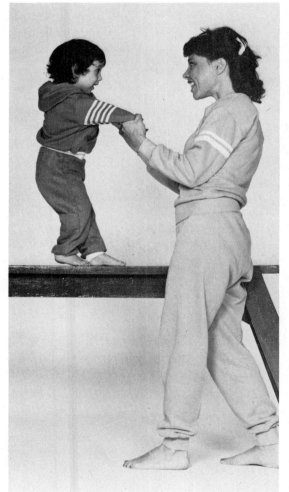

3.
Now place your toddler at one end of the sawhorse or balance beam and have him face that end.

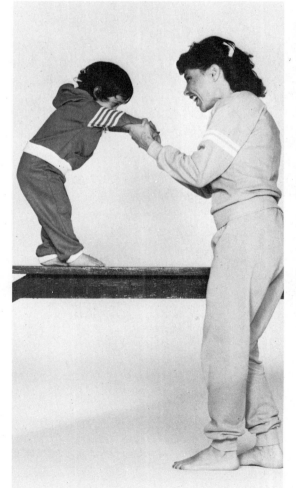

4.
Hold both of your toddler's hands in yours and have him walk back—wards, stepping first with one foot and then the other, all the way across the beam. Tell him which foot he is using each time. Repeat this sequence at least 2 times.

Balance Beam Handstand

There is a daredevil in all of us. Most children love to see the world go upside down—though not for too long a time. Be sure that your toddler's arms are

1.

Place your toddler on a 4-inch-wide balance beam or sawhorse with his hands and feet resting on the beam. Clasp your toddler's hips with both hands, or grasp him around the waist with one hand while holding one leg with the other.

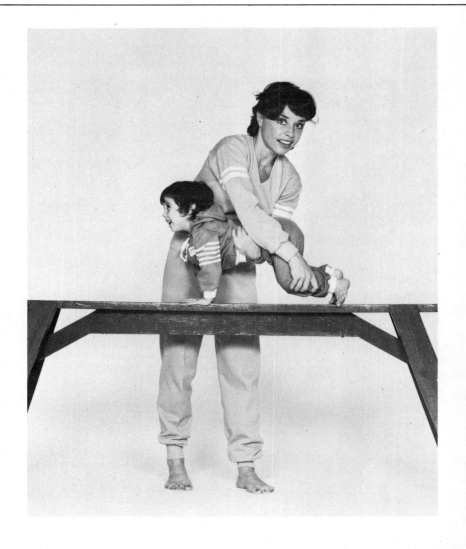

straight during this exercise and that you have a secure grip. Always support your toddler's lower back when raising or lowering his legs. This is an excellent exercise to stimulate circulation and promote a sense of balance and confidence.

2.◆

Raise your toddler's legs, while still supporting him, and then grip both his calves in your hands. With his hands flat on the beam, hold him upside down for a few seconds and then lower him, holding him around the waist as you do so. Repeat the sequence 2 to 4 times.

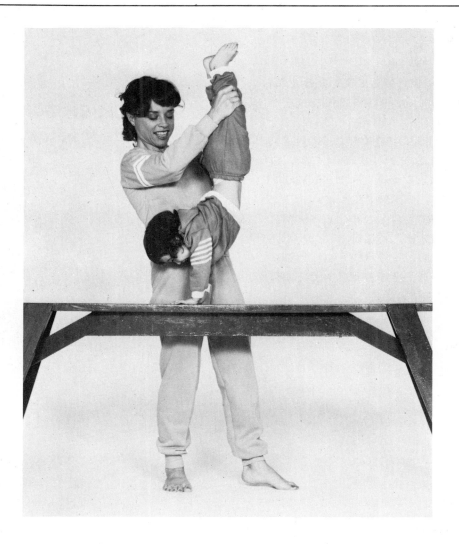

Ramp Walk

The ramp is the most popular piece of equipment at my studio. Toddlers love it. It is extremely versatile and offers them a safe challenge that they can master

1.

Place one end of a 1-foot-wide platform on the floor, with the other end raised and securely propped 1 foot off the floor. Have your toddler walk from the low end to the high end. Be sure to tell your toddler which foot he is using as he goes. After he reaches the high end, have him jump off, landing with both feet. Repeat 4 times.

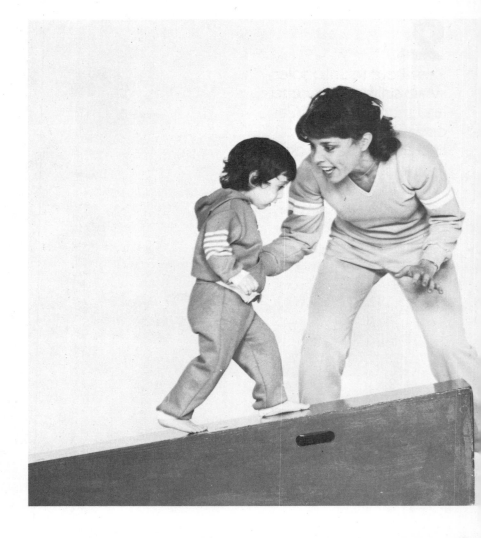

easily. Coordination as well as basic body awareness are easily gained while working with the ramp. If you can't get a proper ramp, a simple platform can be substituted.

2.

Now have your toddler stand on the raised end, facing the low end. Clasp one of his hands in yours, and have him walk down the ramp, telling him which foot he is using as he goes. Repeat 4 times.

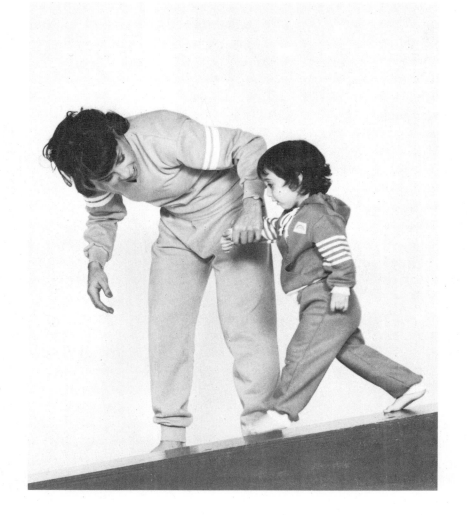

Young Children:
3 to 4 Years

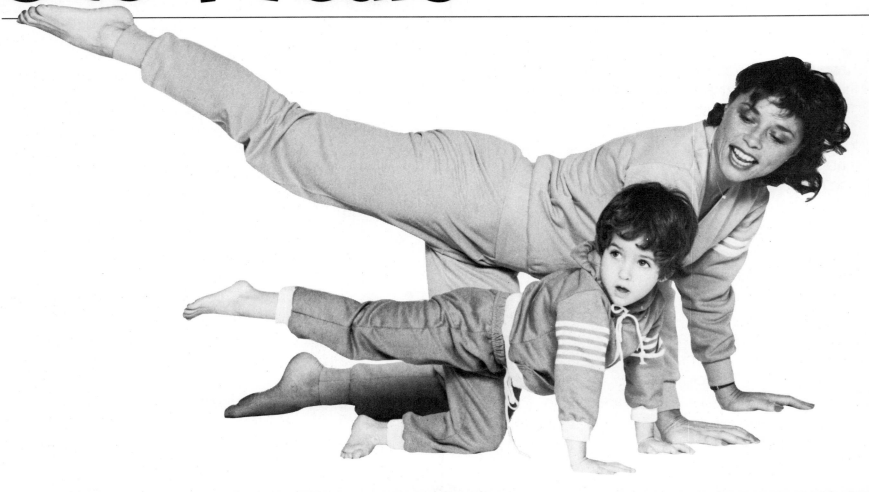

Oh what a joy your three-year-old is (except, perhaps, between 4 and 6 P.M.)! Every day is delightful. True, there are a few tears here and there, but your child's frustration level has evened out, and life, in general, is easier.

You will find that your child is at least fairly well-coordinated by now. Movements that were difficult a few weeks earlier are now easy. Remember those months when you struggled to help him get both feet off the ground when he jumped? Now he's hopping around the room like a kangaroo, as if he'd never had any trouble at all.

You've built a healthy foundation; now is the time to elaborate on it. What does this mean? Be creative. Take each exercise and play with it. Let each movement flow into another. You've been working hard to help your child become strong and well-coordinated. Now that things are easier, make your program more imaginative.

Take exercises from previous sections and from this one and weave a story around them for your child. Create your own program. The following is an example.

One day Inchy Worm decided to go for a walk.
Get down on your tummy and do the Inch Worm exercise across the floor.

On the way, he met Cleo Cat, who was in a very

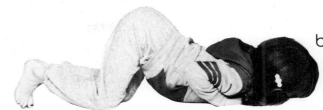

bad mood.
Get down on hands and knees and do the Cat Back exercise 6 times, making hissing noises every time you round your back.

"Why are you in such an angry mood?" said Inchy Worm to Cleo.

"Because of Dorothy Donkey," said Cleo.

"What did she do?"

"She's in an even worse mood than I. She kicked at me!"

"Oh, my," said Inchy. "Let's find out why."

So Cleo Cat climbed up on Inchy's back, and off they went to find Dorothy Donkey.
Do the Inch Worm exercise again.

"There she is," they cried.
Get on hands and knees and do the Donkey Kick exercise 6 times with each leg.

"Dorothy, Dorothy, why are you in such an angry temper?" Inchy and Cleo cried.

"Because I can't fly. I've been watching Mama Bird teach Baby Bird and no matter how hard I try, I can't do it."

"But Dorothy, you're a donkey. You can prance," said Inchy.

"What's that?" asked Dorothy.

"Stand up straight and lift your knees one at a time like this," said Cleo. "That's right, lift one heel off the floor at a time and then the other."

Do the Foot Work exercise 16 times. After 16 repetitions, lift your feet off the floor as if running in place.

"That's wonderful. Now I feel great," said Dorothy. "I'm sorry I kicked at you, Cleo."

"That's all right, Dorothy," said Cleo. "None of us can fly. But we can all try to waddle!"

Do the Duck Walk across the room.

What you just did was an entire series of exercises. All of them were good for various parts of the body. I used only a few exercises here. You can change them, add to them, and create new characters. The three important points are: (1) your child is using his body correctly, thus increasing his strength and coordination; (2) he's using his imagination, thus increasing his intelligence; and (3) you are enjoying each other and sharing a loving experience, thus increasing esteem of yourselves and each other.

Be creative when using the equipment. Try making up a special game with each piece of apparatus, or even combining them. When most people think of hoops, they usually think only of twirling them around their waists. But what a wonderful piece of equipment the hoop is. Children love to jump into and out of hoops. The fact that they must jump over the hoop causes them to jump slightly higher. And because they must focus on placing their bodies in the hoop, they will jump in a more controlled manner. (I have nothing against random jumping, but it's important to learn body control as well.) When the hoops are placed in a pattern, the child must control not only where he is going, but also the speed at which he travels. All in all, hoops are fun, good for developing leg strength, and excellent for coordination.

As your child reaches the age of three and a half, you may notice that he may lose some of his equilibrium–tripping, bumping into things, being a little disjointed. This is natural and will pass. Because you have been exercising your child since birth, he should endure this period more easily than his peers. He may also start to show new and unexplained fears. This, too, is normal and to be expected. For example, he may have a terrible time at this age in coordinating the Ladder Walk, whereas a month ago he wasn't even holding your hand. Just take his hand as if he were starting over again, and work with him until he has mastered it. Repeat this action until he feels secure enough to walk alone again. It will probably not take as long as the first time.

Why do children take this slight step backward? It is my belief that, between the ages of three and three and a half, children are at a slight growth plateau. Suddenly, at three and a half, a growth spurt starts again. Although neither of you can see it, as your child experiences these changes in his size, he is thrown a little off-balance. It is only after he lives in his new size for a while that he becomes comfortable with himself. Be patient, and continue to make the program fun. Your child will grow out of this phase as quickly as he grows out of the new pair of shoes you just bought him.

In general, the time between ages three and four is delightful. You are happy with your child, and your child is happy with you. And what's most fun to watch in your child is the pleasure he gets out of his own body. Louis Bates Ames and Frances L. Ilg of the Gesell Institute of Child Development stated in their book, *Your Three-Year-Old, Friend or Enemy,* "Motor behavior, now relatively secure, can be a source of considerable pleasure to both boys and girls. . . Thus they gallop, jump, walk, and run to music, for the sheer joy of it."

I have included exercises that utilize Frisbees, hoops, a ladder, and a ramp in this section. Use these pieces of equipment and the others mentioned in previous chapters. The time of day you choose for exercise is up to you. I do recommend that your child not be overtired. Use music with a good beat that will help create a happy feeling. Allow your child to choose what he wants to wear. It's a time when your child should feel special. Exercise for perhaps a half hour to 40 minutes one day a week and 15 to 20 minutes the other days. Be creative, and enjoy!

A final note: don't stop exercising with your child after he turns four—create new exercises with the tools I've given you in this book. Remember to make them fun, be sensible with your choices, and maintain your child in a safe and stimulating exercise program.

Inchworm

This highly entertaining way of crossing the room is a great deal of fun. It also builds strength in the entire back, thighs, and shoulders, and enhances coordination.

1.

Lie flat on your stomach, next to each other, with your arms stretched on the floor above your head and your legs stretched straight out on the floor behind you.

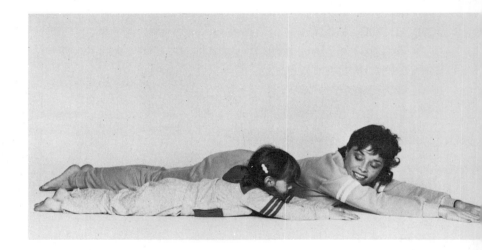

2.

Without separating your legs, raise your bottom up, pulling your knees under you and inching your chest forward so that your arms are bent.

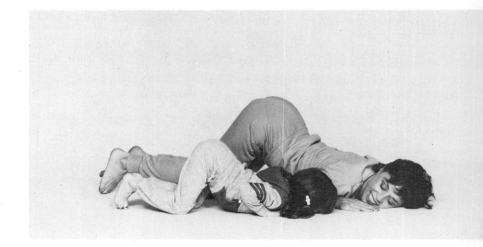

Be sure to keep legs together and chest
on the floor at all times.

3.

Stretch your arms out on
the floor above your
head and let your
stomach come forward
and down onto the floor
so that your body is
straight again. Repeat
the sequence across
the room.

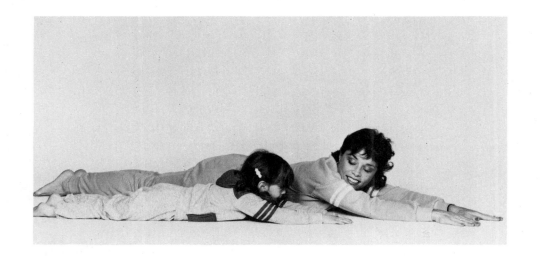

Simple Push-Up

An exercise doesn't have to be difficult to be good. Most children do not have the strength to do a regular push-up, so I modified it. It's better to do

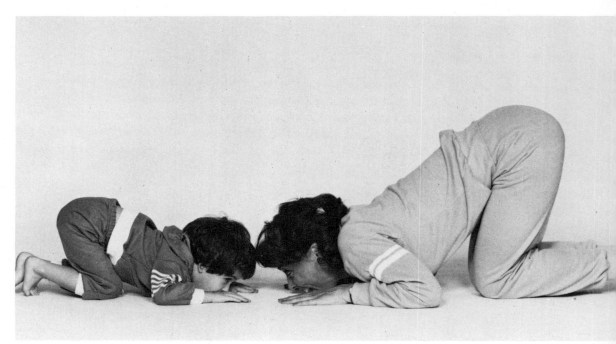

1. Get down on your hands and knees, facing each other or next to each other. Keeping your bottom in the air, bend your arms and lower your chest to the floor.

this simple push-up correctly than the regular one incorrectly. This exercise helps strengthen arm, shoulder, back, and chest muscles.

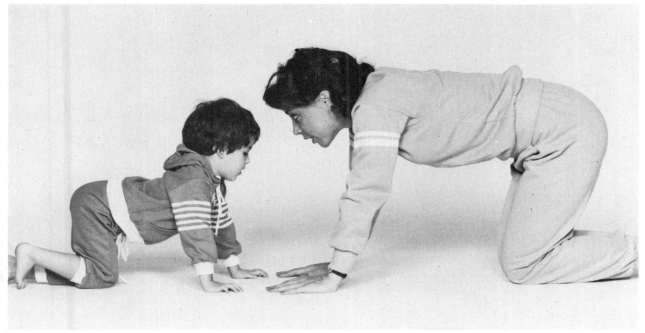

2. Now straighten your arms, pushing your chest away from the floor so that your back is parallel to the floor. Repeat the sequence 8 to 16 times.

Cat Back

Playing an angry cat allows children to exercise their imaginations as well as their abdominal and back muscles. This exercise also enhances lower back

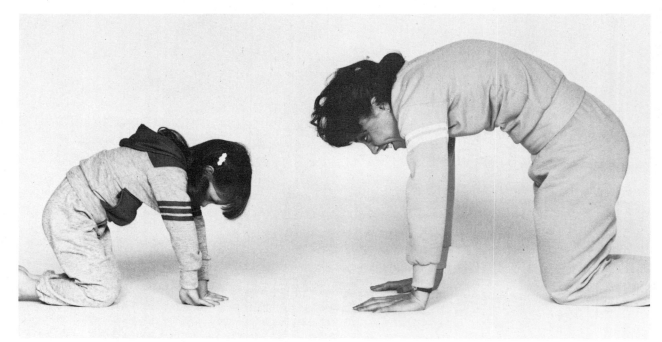

1. Get on your hands and knees. Pull in your stomach and tighten your abdominal muscles, drop your head, and round your back. Hold for 4 seconds.

flexibility. The emphasis should be on the rounding of the back; the second step should be used simply to release muscle tension.

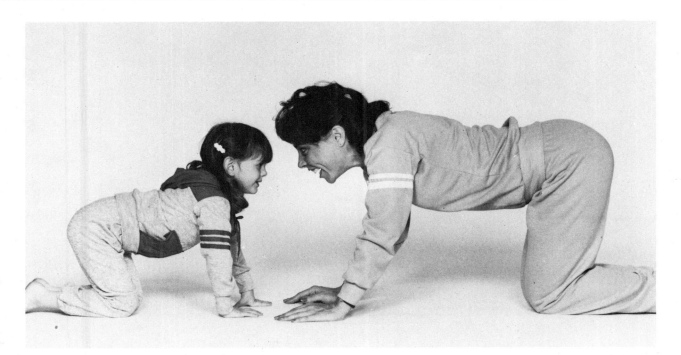

2. Now lift your head and allow your back to sag slightly for 2 seconds. Repeat the sequence 8 times.

Donkey Kick

This is a classic exercise for all ages. It is simple, fun, and excellent for coordination as well as leg (especially upper thigh), buttock, and back strength.

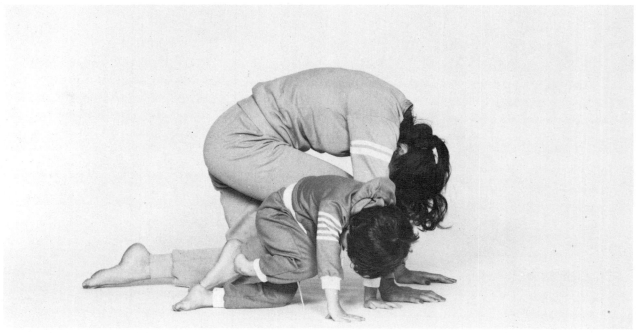

1. Get on your hands and knees next to each other. While keeping your arms straight and your weight evenly distributed between arms and legs, lower your head, round your back, and bring your right knee up under your torso to touch your nose.

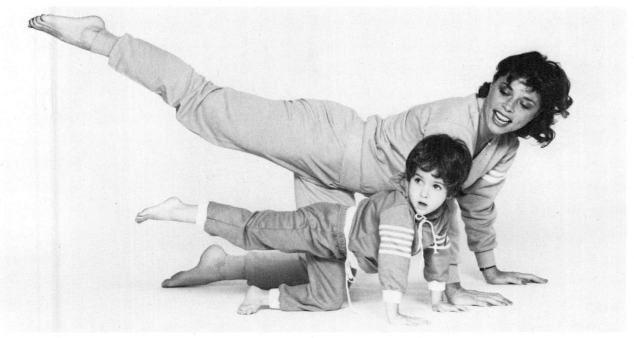

2. Keeping your arms straight, kick your right leg straight out behind you, raising it as high as you can while keeping your hips parallel to the floor. Raise your head at the same time. Repeat the sequence 4 times with each leg.

Foot Work

Feet must carry us correctly and comfortably for an entire lifetime. Our bodies are balanced on them, and they must land and lift as well as support us

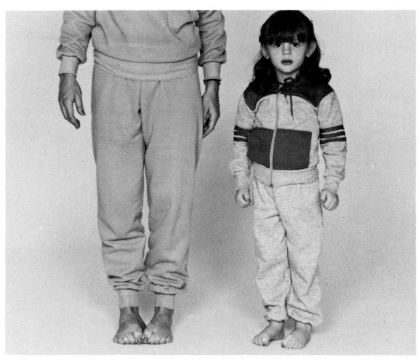

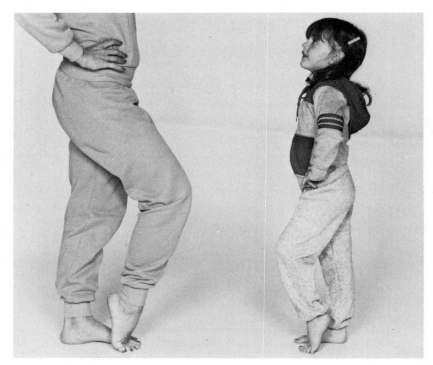

1. Stand with your bare feet flat on the floor. Keeping your legs straight, lean on the outsides of both feet and curl your toes under. Then flatten them down again. Repeat 8 times.

2. Keeping your left foot flat, raise your right heel off the floor, resting it on the ball of the right foot.

properly. Feet spend too many hours in shoes, and the entire foot, including toes, rarely gets a proper workout. In this simple foot exercise, the ankle and calf muscles are exercised as well as the entire foot.

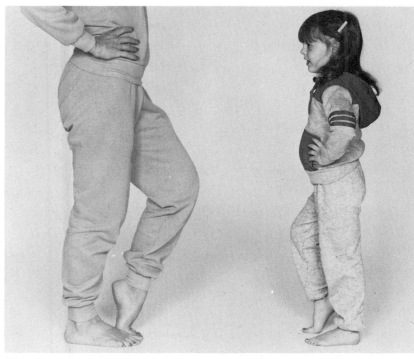

3. While lowering your right heel, lift your left heel off the floor, resting it on the ball of your left foot. Repeat the sequence 8 times.

Pigeon and Duck Walks

The Pigeon Walk looks and sounds simple, but is actually a very difficult coordination exercise. It is excellent for general leg strength, and is especially

1.

Stand next to each other with your feet turned inward, and walk across the room in this manner.

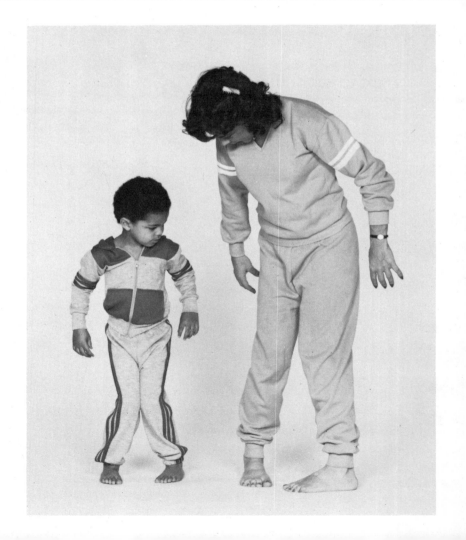

good for children who normally walk with their toes out. The Duck Walk is a much easier exercise, and is good for children who toe in. It is better for coor— dination if done in conjunction with the Pigeon Walk. Try doing the Pigeon Walk for 4 steps, then the Duck Walk for 4 steps, alternating across the room.

2.

Stand next to each other with your feet turned outward, and walk across the room in this manner.

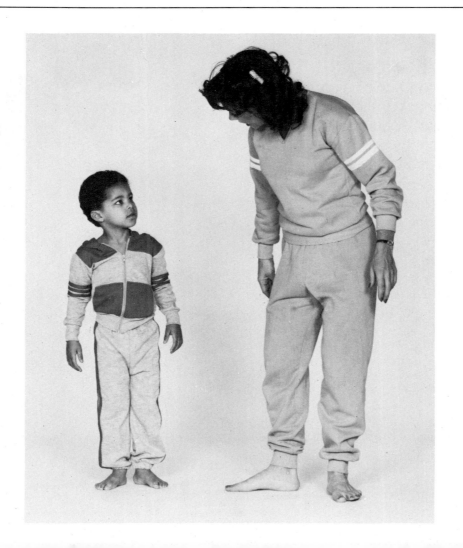

Side-to-Side Knee Bends

This simple exercise is excellent for the entire leg. Knees are gently strengthened as well as the calf, thigh, and ankle muscles, and flexibility of the

1.

Stand next to each other with your legs straight, feet apart and pointing slightly out, and your hands on your hips. Keeping your left leg straight, bend your right knee and place most of your weight on your right leg.

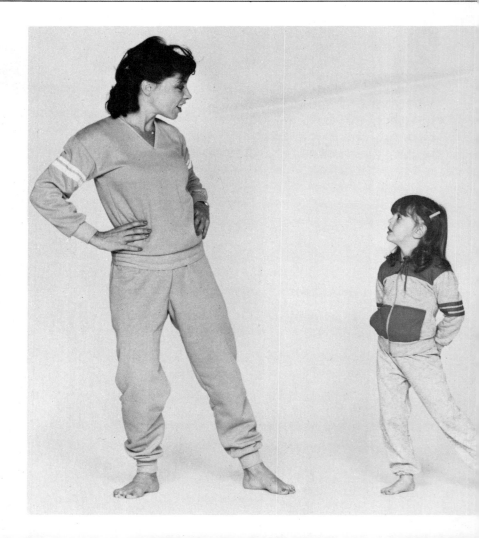

inner leg muscles is enhanced. To make it
more challenging and fun, have your
child do the exercise in tandem with you so
that you both move in the same direction.

2.

Now straighten your right
knee and bend your left
knee, shifting your weight
onto your left leg. Repeat
the sequence 16 times.

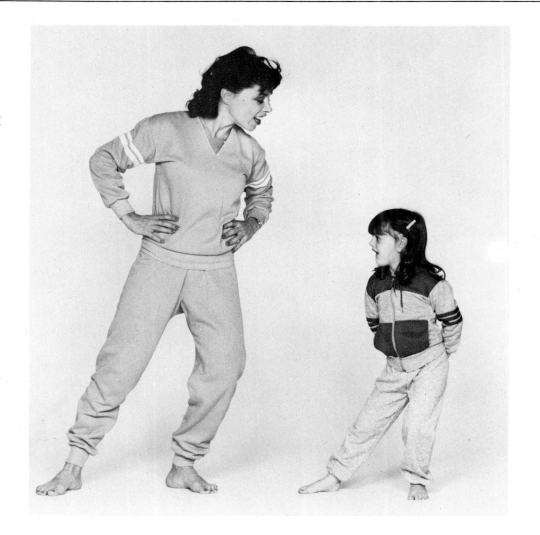

Swing Low, Swing High

The movement in this exercise makes you feel as if you are flying. It is excellent for leg, arm, shoulder, and back strength as well as flexibility and

1.

Stand near each other with your legs straight, feet together and your arms raised above your head.

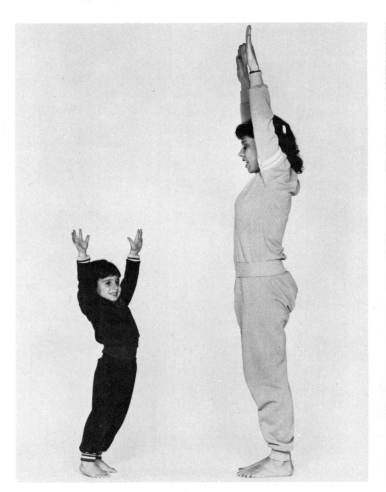

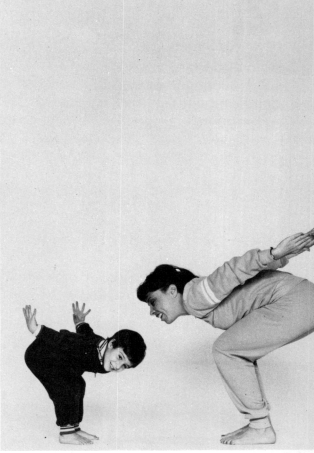

coordination. It also teaches children to move in a smooth, flowing manner rather than a jerky one.

2.

Bending your knees, swing your arms behind you while squatting slightly. Allow your bottom to lift slightly.

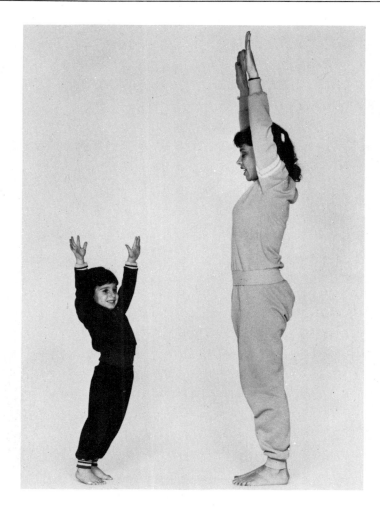

3.

Then swing your arms up again, straight above your head. Repeat the sequence 8 to 16 times.

Push and Pull

Bear in mind while you do this exercise that you are stronger than your child. The object is not to try to push or pull each other off balance but to use each

1.

Stand facing each other with one foot in front of the other and both angled to the left. The outside of your right foot should be placed next to the outside of your child's right foot. Hold each other's right forearm and place your right shoulder against each other's, allowing your child to push against your shoulder as hard as he can. Hold for 4 seconds.

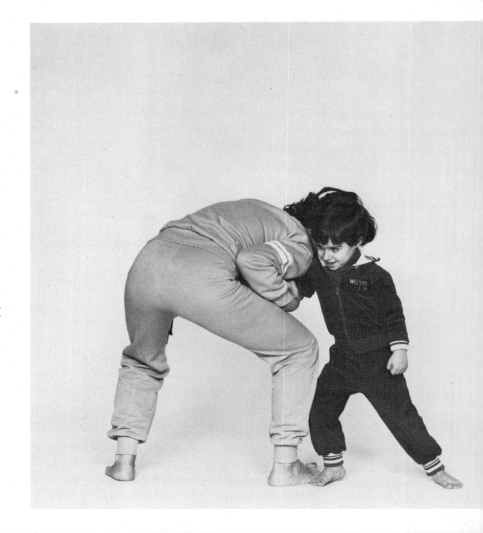

other's weight and strength for gentle resistance. By pushing and pulling slowly against each other's weight, you will gain strength, coordination, and flexibility in the entire body. This exercise is not only fun, it makes children feel powerful, so they enjoy it even more.

2.

Then, still holding each other's forearm, lean outward, placing your weight on your left leg. Allow your child to pull outward as hard as he can. Hold for 4 seconds. Repeat the sequence 4 times with each shoulder.

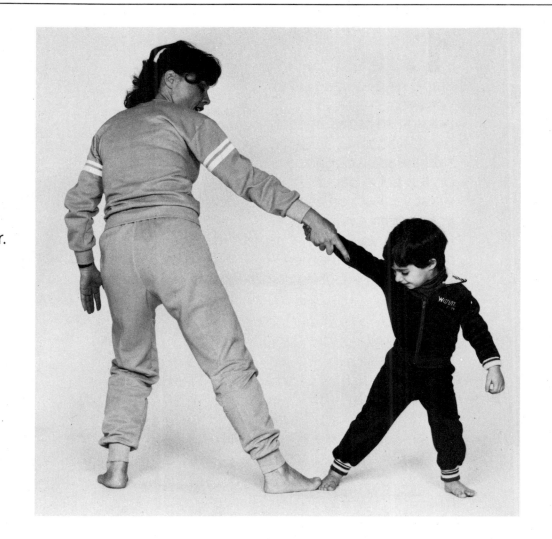

Frisbee Toe Touch

Flexibility, coordination, and fun are the key elements of this exercise. You will be amazed at how many uses a Frisbee has in an exercise program. By placing

1.

Stand next to each other with your feet apart, holding a Frisbee in each hand. Keeping your legs straight and your heels on the floor, bend at the waist so that you touch your left foot with the Frisbee in your right hand. Keep your other hand behind your back.

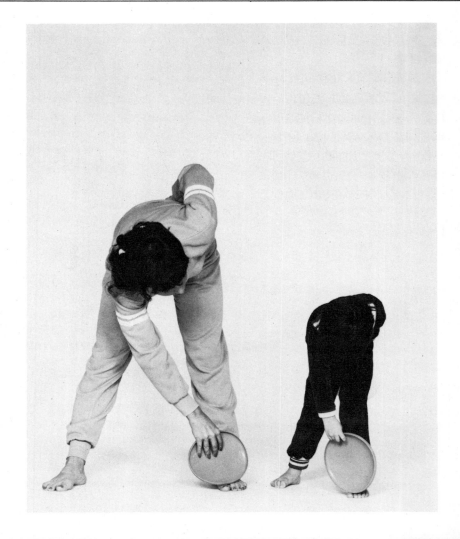

opposite hands (while holding Frisbees) on your feet and telling your child which hand and foot he is using, you further instill in him the knowledge of right and left. At the same time, you are exercising the entire body.

2.

Without standing upright again, touch your right foot with the Frisbee held in your left hand, moving your other hand behind your back. Tell your child which hand and foot he is using each time. Repeat the sequence 8 times.

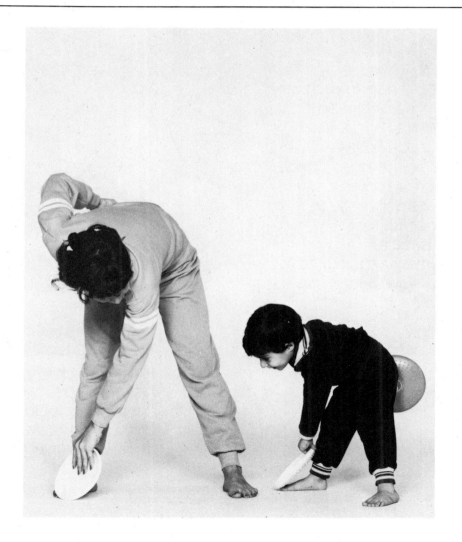

Ramp Rowboat

Arms, shoulders, and the upper back are the areas that gain the most benefit from this exercise. At first, your child may have a few problems with

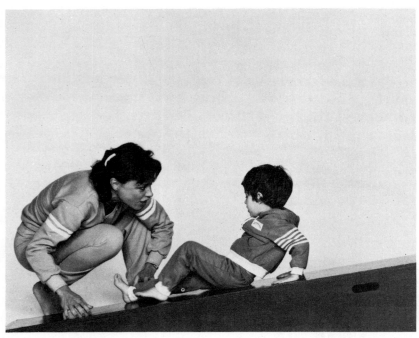

1. Have your child sit on the lowered end of a ramp, facing away from the raised end. His legs should be straight out in front of him, and his hands placed on the ramp behind him.

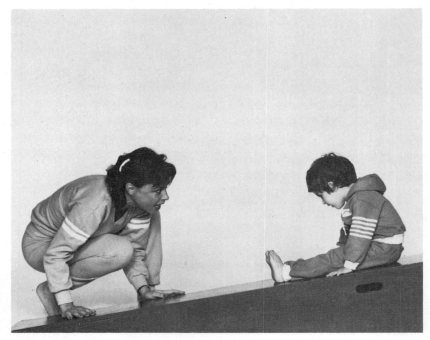

2. Have your child pull his body up between his hands. He should pull himself all the way up the ramp in this manner.

coordination during this exercise, but in time it will become very simple for him. If you can't get a proper ramp, raise and securely prop one end of a platform 1 foot off the floor.

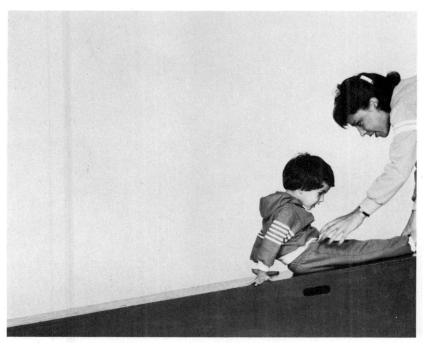

3. Now have your child sit on the raised end of the ramp with his back to the lowered end and his legs facing straight out in front of him. His hands should be placed behind him on the ramp.

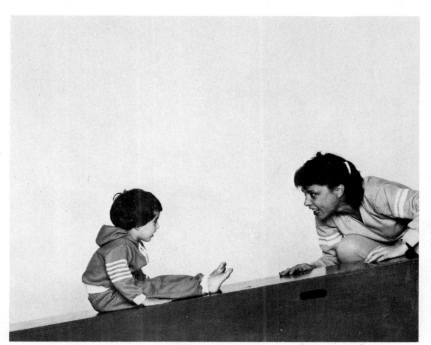

4. Have your child pull his body down the ramp between his hands, and continue in this manner from the raised to the lowered end of the ramp. Repeat the sequence twice.

Ramp Wheelbarrows

This exercise will help increase your child's lower back strength, as well as his arm, shoulder, and chest muscles. It is essential that your child's back not sag

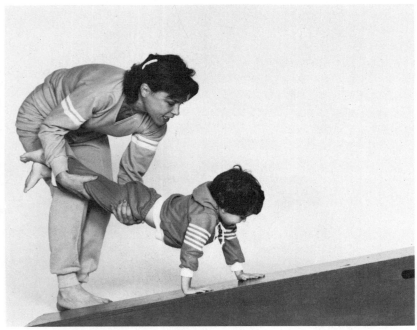

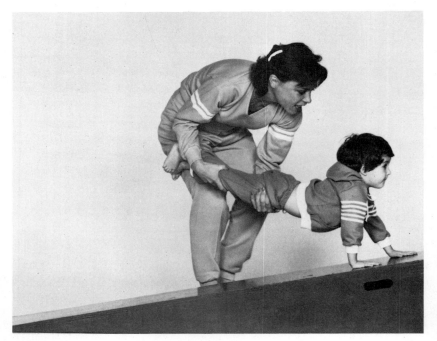

1. Have your child place his hands on the low end of a ramp (or a platform securely propped 1 foot off the floor at one end). Hold his legs up off the floor and support his hips.

2. Have your child walk up the ramp on his hands, supporting him as he goes. Tell him which hand he is placing on the ramp as he goes. Repeat this sequence twice.

when he does it. You must support his hips until his back is strong enough to carry his own weight. As your child gains in strength, you may hold him lower on his legs. Bear in mind that going down the ramp on his hands is harder than going up, since his weight will be thrust forward onto his shoulders and arms.

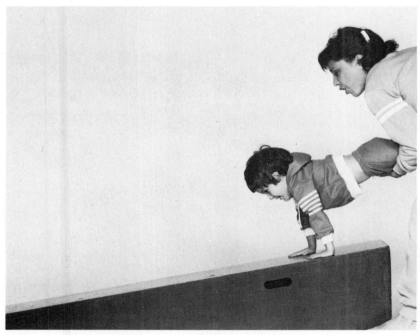

3. Now have your child face down the ramp, placing his hands on the raised end. Hold his legs straight out behind him, supporting his hips so that his back does not sag.

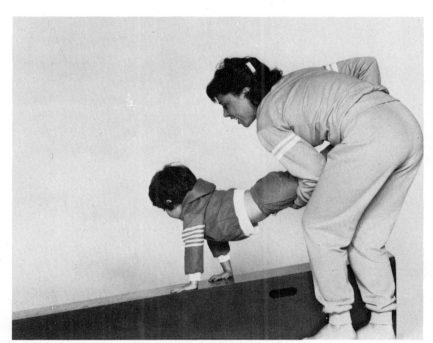

4. Have your child walk down the ramp on his hands. Tell your child which hand he is placing on the ramp as he goes. Repeat this sequence twice.

Hoop Jump

Children love to jump. (If allowed, your child would spend hours jumping up and down on your bed!) Jumping enhances coordination. When a hoop is

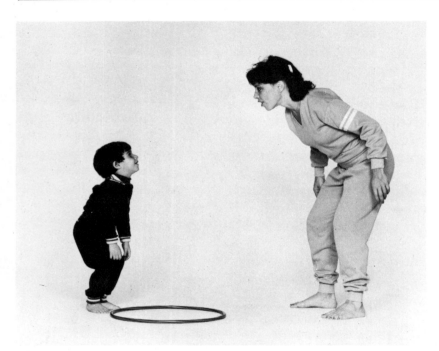

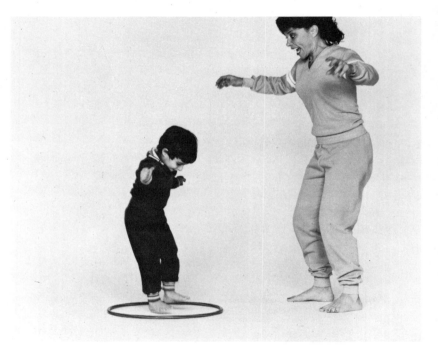

1. Have your child stand outside the rim of a hoop placed on the floor, with his knees slightly bent.

2. Have your child push himself off the floor, straightening his legs and landing inside the hoop with his feet together and his knees bent. Cheer him on as he jumps.

used as a target, concentration as well as balance and coordination are fostered. If your child has difficulty with this exercise at first, help him. Be sure he bends both knees before jumping, and lands on both feet at the same time.

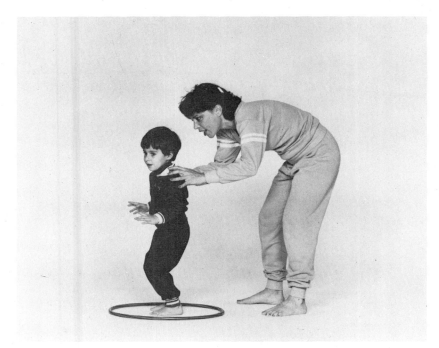

3. Turn your child around so that he faces away from you, and have him bend his knees again in preparation to jump.

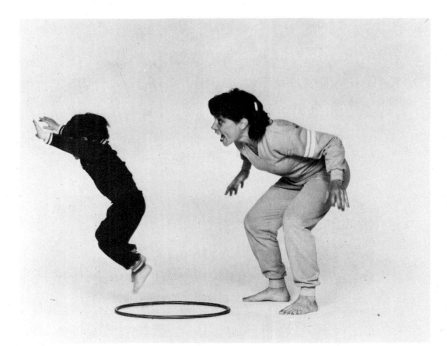

4. Ready, set, go! Your child should push himself off the floor and jump, landing outside the hoop. Repeat the sequence 8 times.

Hopscotch Hoops

Excellent eye-foot coordination is extremely important throughout childhood and beyond, and this exercise greatly enhances it. It is sometimes

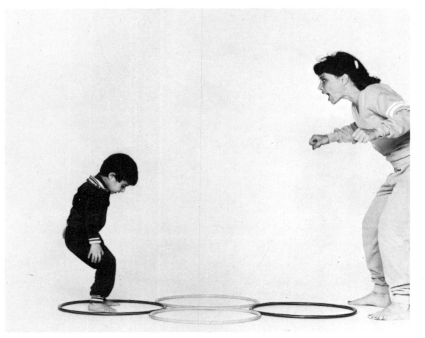

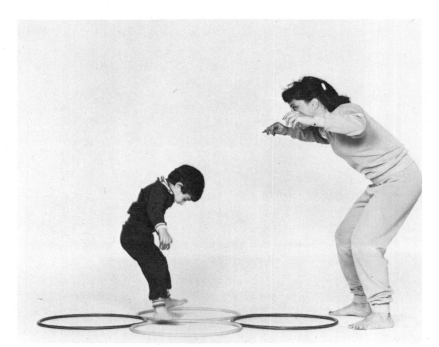

1. Set up 4 hoops on the floor as pictured here. Have your child stand in the first hoop with legs apart and knees slightly bent.

2. Have your child jump into the next two hoops, landing with one foot in each of the hoops that are side by side. Again, his knees should bend when he lands.

necessary to pick your child up and place his feet in the hoops to get him started. But once he gets the idea, there will be no stopping him. After your child is completely familiar with the hopscotch pattern, create different ones with the hoops that offer new challenges for him.

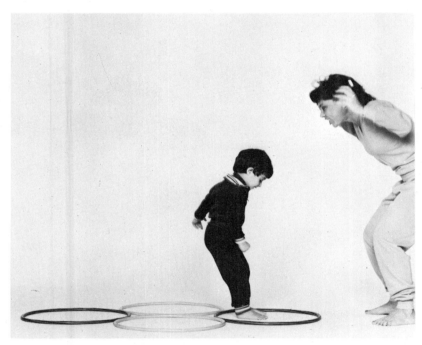

3. Cheering him on, have your child jump a third time, landing in the single hoop at the end with knees bent and feet together. Repeat the sequence 4 times.

Ladder Walk

Ladders can play a versatile part in your exercise program. They can be laid flat to walk on, suspended to hang from, or, as shown here, with one end

1.

Place one end of a ladder on the floor and the other end securely propped 3 feet off the floor. Have your child stand on the lowest rung while you stand by his side, holding his hand.

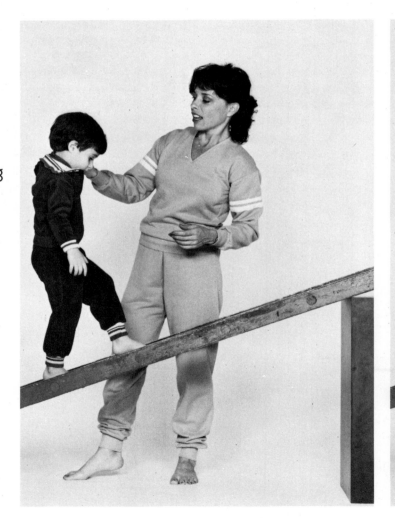
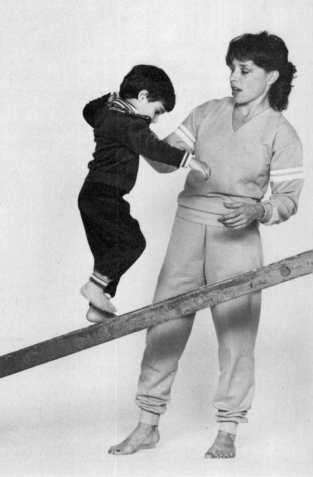

raised and propped to climb on. Leg strength, balance, and coordination are enhanced with this exercise, which is also challenging and fun. Eventually, your child will be able to do it without holding on to you—but always be nearby in case he loses his balance.

2.

Now have your child slowly walk up the ladder, placing one foot at a time on each rung.

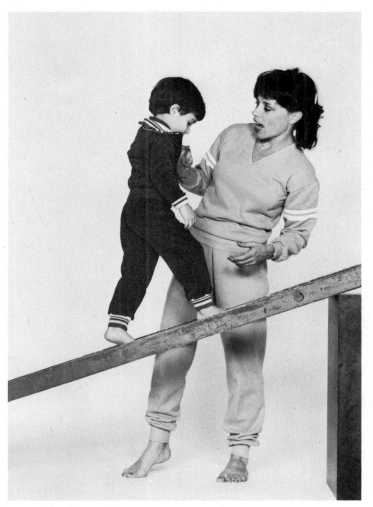

3.

As your child walks from the low end to the raised end of the ladder, have him tell you which foot he is using as he places it on a different rung. Repeat the sequence twice.